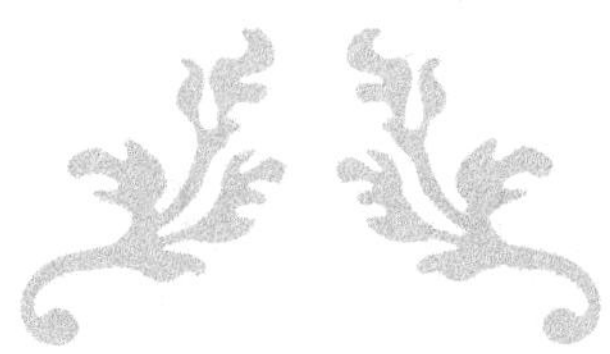

Healthy Meal Planning for Beginners

Three Weekly Meal Plans, 50 Quick and Easy Recipes, and Grocery Lists to Stay Healthy and Lose Weight

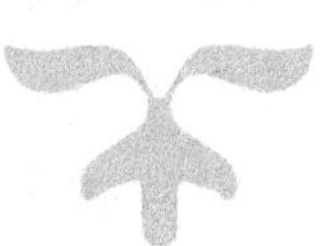

Ami Grace

By reading this document, the reader agrees that under no circumstances is the author responsible for any losses, direct or indirect, that are incurred as a result of the use of the information contained within this document, including, but not limited to, errors, omissions, or inaccuracies.

Table of Content

Introduction

Meal prepping can be compared to an art form. It's something you have to practice and get used to, to ultimately reap the rewards of it. It's a weekly commitment, and failing to plan meals can surely result in you planning to fail, regardless of your efforts.

That is a lesson well learned on my very own journey, as I've tried to reach my goal weight for years. I have spent up to eight years, in fact, trying to lose weight the wrong way. From trying every fad diet for a couple of weeks at a time to obsessing over tracking my macros, trying restrictive diets, and finally, reaching a balance of picking a selection of good food that serves my body, you can surely say I've reached a pivotal point that has set the tone for my healthiest body yet. In truth, eating healthy isn't as difficult as most people think, nor is losing weight. It's all about being well informed, teaching yourself what you should and shouldn't do, and respecting your body in all that it does for you.

I've learned that the biggest problem, both women and men, but especially women, experience with weight loss, is doing it for all the wrong reasons. Approaching a new diet, you should never feel like you're punishing yourself. That is indeed the last thing you should feel like you're doing when it comes to eating healthy. It's not only a means to lose weight, but also to improve your health and sustain it for as long as possible. Since our bodies work like a machine, I quickly recognized the need to nurture it, especially because it's the only one I have.

Filling my body with whole grains or gluten-free alternatives, dairy-free products, a variety of vegetables, fruit, nuts, seeds, healthy sources of protein, good fats, and a range of superfoods, has shaped a healthier body, mental well-being, and even my emotional relationship with food. Now, instead of restricting myself, I choose whole foods and count the calories of each meal to ensure I meet my daily nutrition needs, steering away from eating empty calories either, overeating or restricting myself too much. In the past few months, I have specifically found a lot of value in prepping my meals on a Sunday and Wednesday evening. It has allowed me to maintain discipline each week by visiting the grocery store instead of ordering in, preparing meals I like, and learning new and exciting recipes I can integrate into each new week. Meal prepping has served as a big tool on my journey towards reaching a healthy relationship with good food and losing my unwanted weight.

Depending on your reason or goal, meal prepping can come in handy for all those busy days at the office, home, school, or wherever you may find yourself. It can improve your diet, save time, and aid in your weight-loss, which is one of the biggest reasons why I integrated it into my diet. That is exactly why I felt inspired to write this book, which includes 50 healthy, meal prepping, and inspirational recipes to help you get started.

Since losing weight or getting healthier are both processes that take time, it's quite necessary to discover what works for you. Prepping your meals once or twice a week is a great effort to resist the possible loss of motivation on your diet or journey to living a more wellness-inspired lifestyle.

Chapter 1: Why Do You Need to Plan Your Diet?

Since we live in a fast-paced world, many of us forget to slow down, which is why it is necessary to ask ourselves, what suits our lifestyle best? If you're not into following fad diets, or perhaps any other diet that you feel requires too much effort, then it's best to start with a basic healthy and balanced diet.

Consistency and discipline are two traits that will go hand in hand in creating a successful meal planning experience. Given that most people's goals are to lose weight, you can just imagine why planning your daily meals is so important.

Golden Rules of Healthy Eating

#1 Master your ingredient list.

You can decide on your recipes for the week and create a smart grocery list. Now, without getting overwhelmed, you can divide your list into two parts. The first part is for your pantry, which includes ingredients you can stock up on once a month instead of weekly. The second part is weekly ingredients that typically belong in your refrigerator. Simplifying your weekly ingredient list by only focusing on fresh foods is much more convenient. In this way, your grocery list will be kept simple, preventing you from running out of ingredients.

#2 Focus on fiber.

When the average individual approaches dieting, they tend to remove ingredients or even food groups altogether from their diets. One food group, in particular, are carbohydrates, and I don't know about you, but aren't carbs considered one of the simplest and best sources of fiber? That's why quitting a food group altogether is never the answer. Your body needs a balance between all food groups to thrive optimally and to survive. Adding adequate sources of fiber to your diet can help stabilize your blood sugar levels, support healthy digestion, and ensure that your gut remains healthy. Adding a source of fiber, whether it's a carbohydrate, fruit, vegetable, or protein to each meal, will also help promote effective and sustainable weight loss, and prevent your body from holding on to water weight and body fat.

#3 Fill up on protein at each meal.

When it comes to staying full and targeting body fat, the best thing you can do is eat more animal protein. Sources of animal protein are complete proteins, containing nine essential amino acids, all of which aid in maintaining and restructuring the protein compounds in your body. Adding protein to each meal also keeps you fuller for longer and doesn't get stored in the body as fat. Instead, it gets used as slow-energy releasing sources of fuel, which promotes weight loss, decreased appetite, improved muscle restoration, and functioning, and a healthy body. Some of the best sources of complete proteins include chicken, eggs, grass-fed beef, seafood, and pasture-raised lamb.

#4 Fat is good for your health and weight loss.

There's a common myth about eating fat and how it only causes you to gain weight. However, it's not true. Healthy fats, including monounsaturated, polyunsaturated, and even a small quantity of saturated fats, are good for you and the functioning of your brain. On the other hand, anything processed, the worse being trans fat, must be avoided. Healthy fats can be added to meals to improve the healthy functioning of your body, support your cells, and do wonders for weight loss.

#5 Hydrate properly.

Is there a right way to hydrate wrong? Yes... It's called not hydrating at all because many individuals like to drink two glasses of water and call it a day, which is not going to support the amount of fluid your body needs to function properly. Without the adequate intake of water, your body can't perform proper digestive functions, nor clear your blood of waste, which could create a danger zone for your organs, cells, and bodily processes. A dehydrated body can result in blood circulation, cell functionality, and regeneration issues, and prevent the body from absorbing nutrients properly. It is recommended that adults consume 50 oz to 100 oz of water every day.

The Formula for Calculating Daily Calorie Intake

To calculate your daily calorie intake, keep in mind that 1,000 kilocalories = 1 calorie.
To establish how many calories you eat during the day, you can make use of the calorimeter. It is a tool used by scientists and nutritionists to calculate the calories in all types of food. Since the total number of calories you consume plays a big role in weight loss, it's necessary to know how much your body needs to sustain itself, and ultimately, to lose weight. Many apps are made available to calculate your calorie intake.

Alternatively, to calculate your calorie intake, you have to calculate your basal metabolic rate (BMR + activity level).

Your BMR refers to the total number of energy expenditure your body needs to support the proper functioning, including blood circulation, breathing, brain, and nerve functioning, as well as body temperature regulation.

After you've established your BMR, you should calculate your activity level. For this calculation, you need to calculate your exercise level and your non-exercise activity thermogenesis (NEAT).

By calculating these two activity expenditures, you will be able to establish the total number of calories you burn during exercise, and throughout your entire day performing daily activities.

Daily calorie intake = BMR + NEAT + burned calories during exercise.

#1 BMR formula

BMR (kcal / day) = 10 * **weight** (kg) + 6.25 * height (cm) − 5 * age (y)

#2 Activity calculation

Activity calorie expenditure can be calculated by sport's devices, like sports watches or tracked by cardio machines in the gym.

How to Use This Book

The Healthy Meal Planning for Beginners book serves as a guide to help you achieve a balanced relationship and daily disciplined routine with food.
It includes three different 7-day meal plans included in this guide, which means you have 21 days of healthy meal planning recipes to choose from. Since it only takes three weeks to form a new habit, this guide is perfect for doing just that. It supports the idea of remaining disciplined in the action you take to achieve your goals, which can transcend into something more satisfactory and attainable.

It is also designed with the necessary information for you to draw up meal plans that suit your week and are tailored to your own needs. By calculating your calorie needs, and reviewing the recipes, you can pick breakfast, lunch, dinner, snacks, and dessert recipes that fit together and meets the number of calories you require daily to sustain your body's natural calorie needs, as well to exert energy by exercising or performing daily tasks and activities.

As an example: If your daily recommended calorie intake is 1,600 calories (BMR), your average activity level is 400 calories (NEAT), and the calories you burn during exercise is 300, then you need to consume 2,300 calories on average daily.

To consume 2,300 calories, you can choose the following meals:

- Breakfast - 600 calories
- Snack - 250 calories
- Lunch - 600 calories
- Dinner - 550 calories
- Snack - 300 calories

This book includes 50 simple meal-planning recipes, all of which include calories per single serving to simplify setting up your own personal meal plant. The recipes are also complete with shopping lists, simplifying the entire process of meal planning for you.

Chapter 2: 50 Recipes for Meal Prepping

Breakfast Recipes

#1 Egg Salad Sandwiches

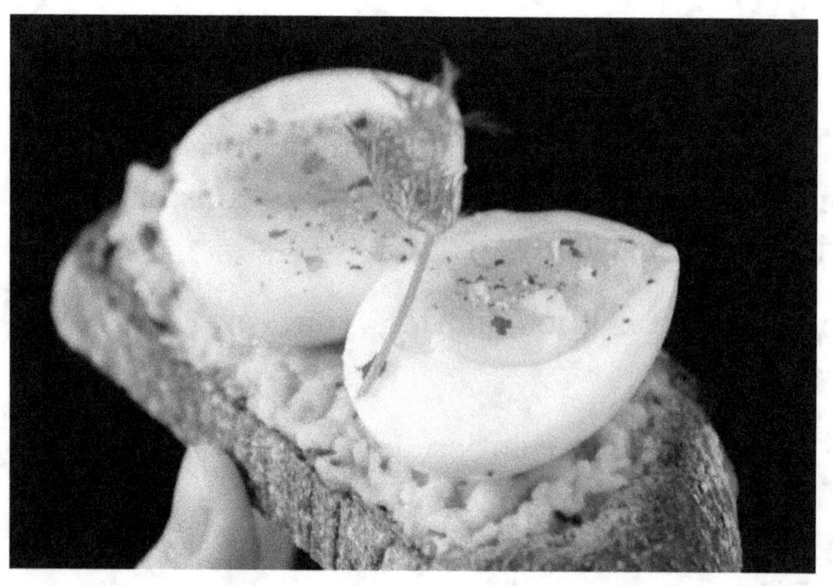

Serving size: 4 Servings

Calories: 250 (1 serving)

Preference: Gluten-free, dairy-free, sugarless

Duration: 10 minutes

Ingredients:

- 4 eggs (boiled)
- 8 slices gluten-free bread
- 2 cups of green onion (diced)
- 2 stalks of celery (chopped)
- 4 large lettuce leaves
- 4 tsp of hummus (plain)
- Himalayan salt and black pepper

Directions:

1. Peel and slice the boiled eggs in four to five pieces each, and set it aside.
2. Mix the prepped green onion, celery, hummus, and black pepper in a bowl.
3. Spread the onion-hummus mixture onto the four slices of bread.
4. Place one sliced boiled egg on each slice of bread with the onion-hummus mixture.
5. Add Himalayan salt and extra black pepper on top. Place a lettuce leaves on each prepped slice, and place another slice of bread on top. Slice the sandwiches in half or quarters, and seal them in plastic wrap or Ziploc bags. Place them in the refrigerator for up to three days.

#2 Peanut Butter Bite

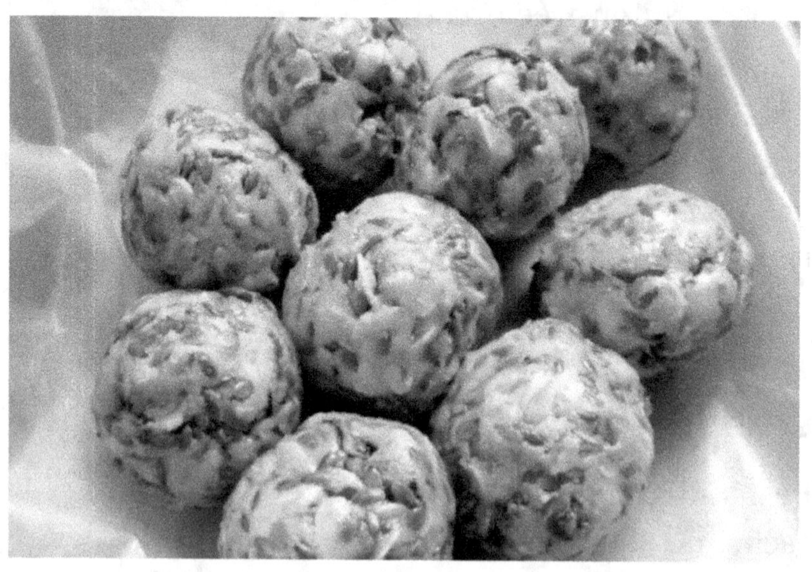

Serving size: 12 bites - 4 servings (3 per serving)

Calories: 500 calories (1 serving)

Preference: Gluten-free, vegetarian

Duration: 10 minutes

<u>Ingredients:</u>

- 1 cup of rolled oats (gluten-free)
- ½ cup of peanut butter (smooth)
- ½ cup of chocolate chips
- ½ cup of flax seeds (ground)
- 2 tbsps. of sweetener (agave nectar or honey)

<u>Directions:</u>

1. Combine the rolled oats, peanut butter, chocolate chips, flax seeds, and sweetener of choice in a bowl.
2. Place the mixture in the refrigerator for 15 minutes
3. Remove the mixture from the refrigerator and roll the dough into 12 individual bite-sized balls. Store in the refrigerator for five to seven days in an airtight container.

#3 Breakfast Burritos

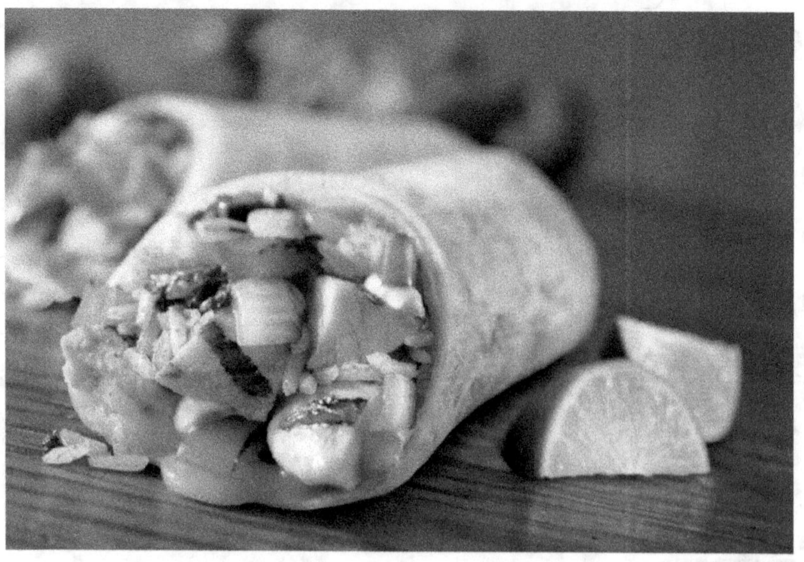

Serving size: 4 servings

Calories: 420 (1 serving)

Preference: None

Duration: 30 minutes

Ingredients:

- 6 eggs (large)
- 4 whole wheat tortillas (large)
- 1 cup of black beans
- 1 cup of mozzarella cheese (grated)
- ½ cup of cherry tomatoes (halved)

- 1 jalapeno (halved)
- ½ onion (diced)
- 1 tbsp of olive oil
- 1 tbsp of thyme
- ½ tsp of black pepper

Directions

1. Heat a large, non-stick pan with 1 tbsp. of olive oil over medium heat.
2. Add the diced onions and cook for 1-2 minutes.
3. Add the black beans, cherry tomatoes, and jalapeno. Cook for 1-2 minutes.
4. Beat the eggs in a medium bowl, add the thyme and black pepper.
5. Pour the egg mixture into the pan and use a spatula to move it around until you've reached a cooked scrambled consistency, ensuring the ingredients are combined well.
6. Spread the grated mozzarella cheese all over the scramble and allow it to melt.
7. Switch off the heat, plate the tortillas, and divide the bean-scramble between four plates.
8. Fold the burritos carefully, ensuring all corners of the burrito is covered.
9. Wrap the burritos in foil, and store it in an airtight container for up to three days. Alternatively, store the foil-covered burritos in the freezer for two to three weeks.

#4 Get-Your-Greens Sweet Potato Frittata

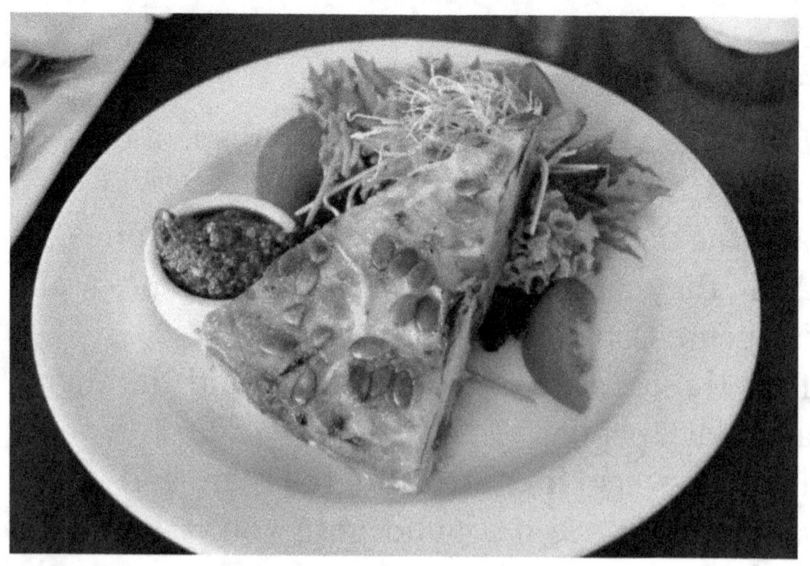

Serving size: 4 servings
Calories: 325 (1 serving)
Preference: Gluten-free, sugarless
Duration: 30 minutes

Ingredients:

- 6 eggs (large)
- 2 cups of sweet potato (washed, peeled, and cubed)
- 2 cups of kale (washed and chopped)
- ¼ cup of mozzarella cheese (grated)
- ½ red onion (diced)
- 2 tbsp of olive oil
- 2 cloves of garlic (minced)

- ½ tsp of black pepper
- 1 tsp of Himalayan salt

Directions:

1. Preheat the oven to 350 degrees Fahrenheit.
2. In a medium bowl, beat the eggs, salt, and black pepper.
3. On a non-stick baking sheet, place the cubed sweet potatoes and drizzle 1 tbsp of olive oil on top. Place the baking sheet in the oven and cook for 10 minutes.
4. Remove the sweet potatoes from the oven.
5. In a pan, over medium heat, cook the kale, diced onion, and minced garlic in 1 tbsp of olive oil for 3 minutes. Add the cooked sweet potato to the pan and mix everything.
6. Sprinkle mozzarella cheese on top and switch off the stove.
7. Spray a medium casserole dish with cooking spray. Transfer the pan ingredients to the casserole dish, and pour the egg mixture over it until everything is leveled.
8. Place the casserole dish in the oven, and bake it for 10 minutes.
9. Once done, allow it to cool down. Slice it into four servings and place it in an airtight container for the perfect on-the-go breakfast. Store in the fridge for three to four days.

#5 Banana-Blueberry Protein Muffins

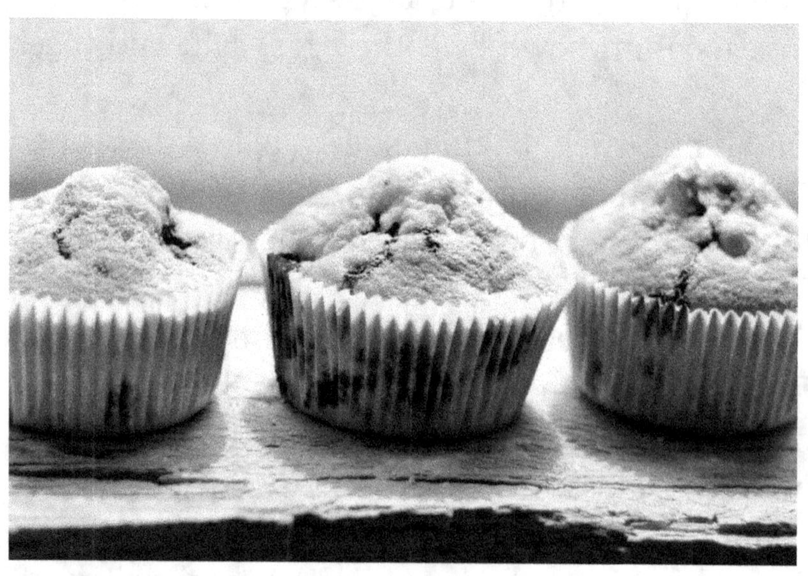

Serving size: 8 muffins (2 x 4 servings)

Calories: 200 (1 serving)

Preference: Dairy-free

Duration: 30 minutes

Ingredients:

- 2 eggs
- 2 bananas (ripe)
- ½ cup of blueberries
- ¾ cup of peanut butter (or nut butter of choice)
- ¼ cup of honey
- ½ tbsp of vanilla extract
- ¼ tsp of baking soda

Directions:

1. Preheat the oven to 400 degrees Fahrenheit.
2. Spray a small-medium muffin pan with cooking spray.
3. Add eggs, bananas, peanut butter, honey, vanilla extract, and baking soda in a blender. Blend until you've reached a smooth texture.
4. Add the blueberries to the mixture.
5. Divide the mixture between eight muffin cups ¾ full.
6. Bake the muffins for 15 minutes in the oven, and allow it to cool down after that.
7. Place the muffins in an airtight container for up to five days.

#6 Pumpkin Glow Smoothie

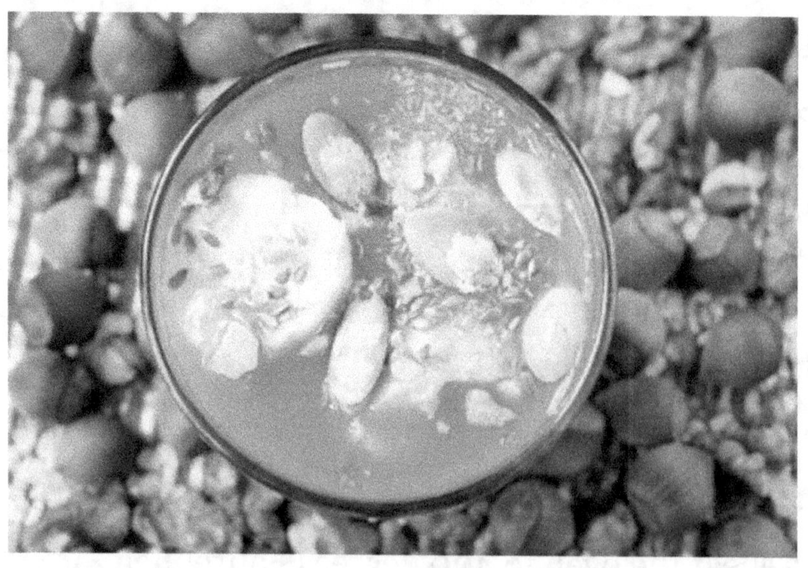

Serving size: 4 servings

Calories: 225 (1 serving)

Preference: Gluten-free, vegetarian

Duration: 5 minutes

Ingredients:

- 8 tbsps. of pure pumpkin (canned)
- 8 tbsps. of Greek yogurt
- ½ cup of almond milk
- 4 bananas (frozen)
- 2 tsp of honey
- 4 tsp of chia seeds
- ½ tsp of cinnamon
- ½ tsp of nutmeg
- 1 cup of ice

Directions:

1. Blend the ingredients all together for 1 to 2 minutes. Pause halfway to scrape down the sides of the blender. Blend until you've reached a smooth texture.

2. Serve cold with 1 tsp of chia seeds per serving, or refrigerate in airtight mason jars for up to two days.

#7 Sweet Vitamin-Kick Walnut Oatmeal

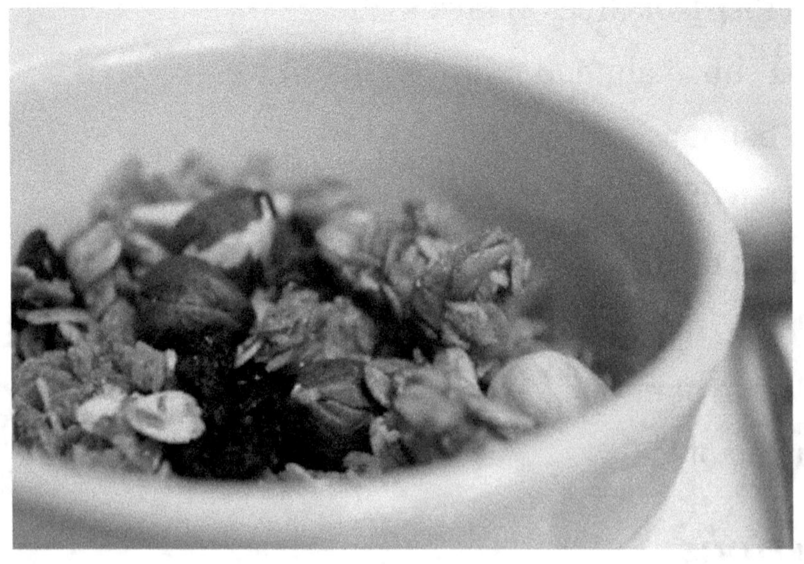

Serving size: 4 servings

Calories: 500 (1 serving)

Preference: Dairy-free, vegetarian

Duration: 30 minutes

Ingredients:

- 2 cups of rolled oats
- 2 cups of almond milk
- 2 cups of pineapple (chopped)
- 2 eggs (large)
- ½ cup of honey
- 1 cup of walnuts (chopped)
- 2 tsp of vanilla extract
- ½ tsp of kosher salt
- 1 piece of ginger (grated)

Directions:

1. Preheat the oven to 400 degrees Fahrenheit.
2. Mix the rolled oats, pineapple, grated ginger, walnuts, and salt in a bowl.
3. Once mixed, divide the oatmeal mixture into four separate ramekins.
4. In another bowl, combine the almond milk, vanilla extract, and honey.
5. Pour ¼ of the wet mixture over the oatmeal and pineapple mixture in ramekin dishes.
6. Place the ramekins on a baking sheet, and allow the oats to bake for 20 minutes.
7. Serve the oatmeal with the milk-honey syrup on the side, or cover the ramekin dishes with plastic, and store it in the refrigerator for up to three days. Place the milk-honey syrup in a separate airtight container, and serve it with the oatmeal whenever you like.

#8 Blueberry Coconut Chia Jars

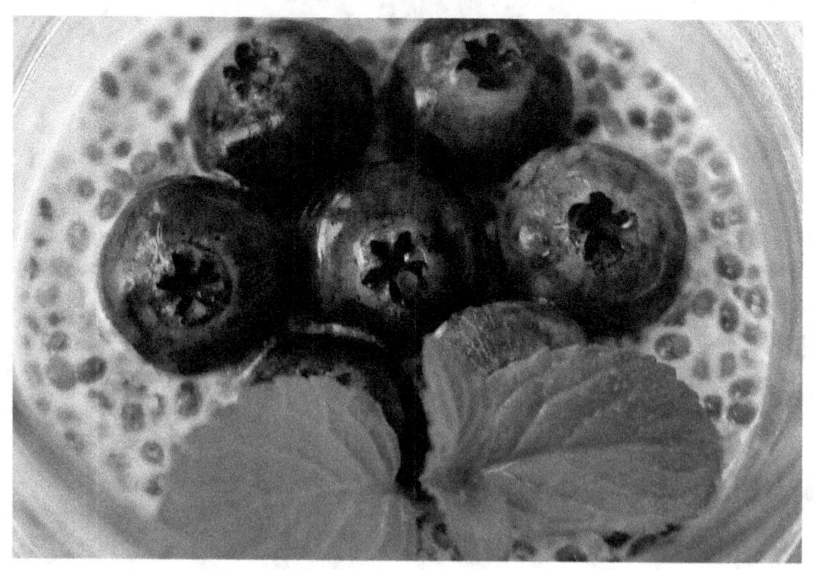

Serving size: 4 servings

Calories: 300 (1 serving)

Preference: Gluten-free, dairy-free, vegetarian

Duration: 10 minutes (refrigerate overnight)

<u>*Ingredients:*</u>

- 2 cups of rolled oats (gluten-free)
- 3 cups of coconut milk
- 1 cup of blueberries
- 4 tbsp. of chia seeds
- 4 tbsp. of honey
- 1 tsp of lemon zest
- ¼ tsp of cinnamon

<u>*Directions:*</u>

1. In four 16-oz mason jars, add ½ cup of oats, 1 tbsp. of honey, 1 tbsp. of chia seeds, and a ¾ cup of coconut milk.

2. Stir all of the ingredients together in each jar, and refrigerate it overnight.

3. Serve with a ¼ tsp of lemon zest, cinnamon, and blueberries on top.

#9 Honey Granola and Greek Yogurt

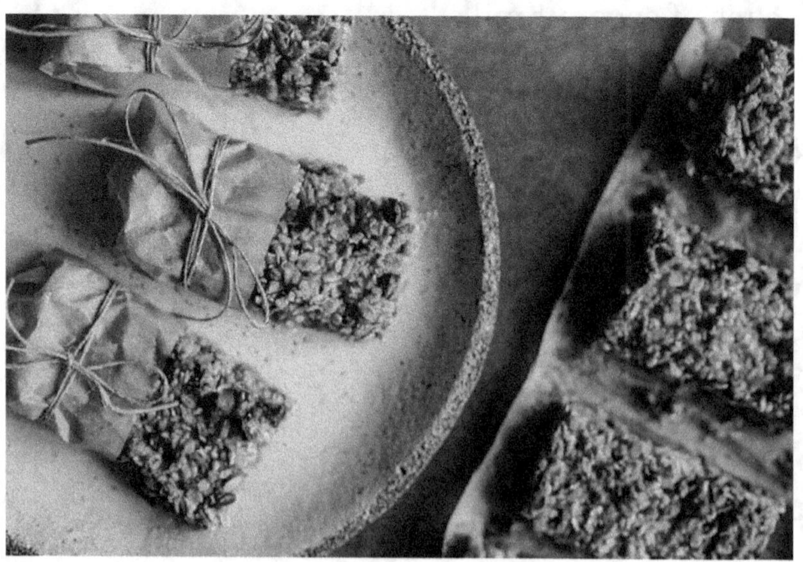

Serving size: 4 servings

Calories: 650 calories (1 serving)

Preference: Gluten-free, vegetarian

Duration: 25 minutes

Ingredients:

- 4 cups of rolled oats (gluten-free)
- 1 cup of mixed nuts (chopped)
- ½ cup of raisins
- 1 tbsp. of cinnamon
- ¼ tsp of salt
- 1-½ cup of honey
- 4 cups of Greek yogurt
- 2 cups of mixed berries

Directions:

1. Combine the oats, mixed nuts, raisins, salt, and cinnamon in a bowl.
2. Preheat the oven to 300 degrees Fahrenheit.
3. Line a baking sheet with parchment paper, and place the granola mixture on top, spreading it evenly.
4. Drizzle the honey on top of the granola mixture, and put it in the oven to bake for 20 minutes.
5. Remove the granola from the oven and allow it to cool down.
6. Once cooled, place it in a glass jar, and store it at room temperature for a few weeks.
7. Serve the granola with Greek yogurt, mixed berries, and an added glaze of honey.

#10 Tropical Smoothie Bowl

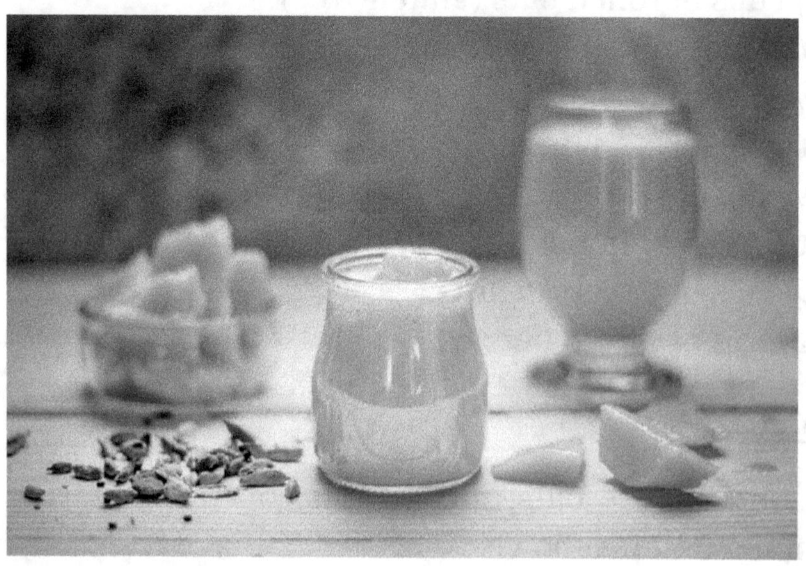

Serving size: 4 servings

Calories: 260 (1 serving)

Preference: Gluten-free, dairy-free, Vegetarian, Vegan

Duration: 5-10 minutes

Ingredients:

- 2 bananas (frozen)
- 2 cups of almond milk
- 2 cups of mango (frozen)
- 1 cup of pineapple (frozen)
- ½ cup of blanched almonds
- 2 Kiwis (sliced)
- ½ fresh mango (sliced)
- ½ cup of blueberries

Directions:

1. Add the frozen bananas, frozen mango, almond milk, and pineapple to a blender, and blend it for 1 minute, or until it reaches a smooth consistency.
2. To serve, divide the smoothie mixture into four separate bowls. To store, refrigerate in four different mason jars for up to two days. When serving, decorate the smoothie bowl with sliced kiwis, fresh mango, blueberries, and blanched almonds.
3. Serve cold.

Lunch Recipes

#1 Creamy Tofu Salad

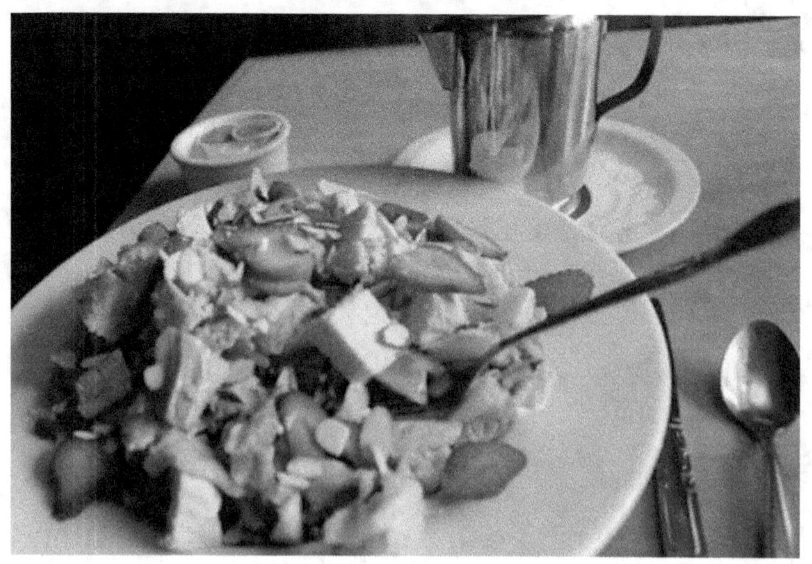

Serving size: 4 servings

Calories: 250 (1 serving)

Preferences: Gluten-free, Vegetarian

Duration: 25 minutes

Ingredients:

- 1 lb. soft tofu, cut into 1/2 thick triangles.
- 8 romaine lettuce leaves
- 3 celery stalks (chopped)
- 1 apple (cored and chopped)
- 1 cup of strawberries
- ½ cup of pecan nuts (roasted)
- 1/4 inch of oil
- Dressing: ¾ cup of Greek yogurt, 2 tbsps. of water, 1 tbsp. of apple cider vinegar, 1 tbsp. of lemon juice, 1 tbsp. of honey, 1tsp of poppy seeds, ¼ tsp of pepper.

Directions:

1. Heat about 1/4 inch of oil in a skillet over medium heat. Fry the tofu cubes on all sides until golden brown, remove to drain on a paper towel.
2. Place the chopped apple in a bowl with lemon juice.
3. Divide all the salad ingredients, including the tofu, seasoned apple, celery, strawberries, pecan nuts, and romaine lettuce into four mason jars.
4. Seal the jars with lids and place them in the refrigerator until ready to serve. The salads can be stored in the refrigerator for up to three days. Serve the dressing once you are ready to eat the salad separately.

#2 Chicken Avocado Burritos

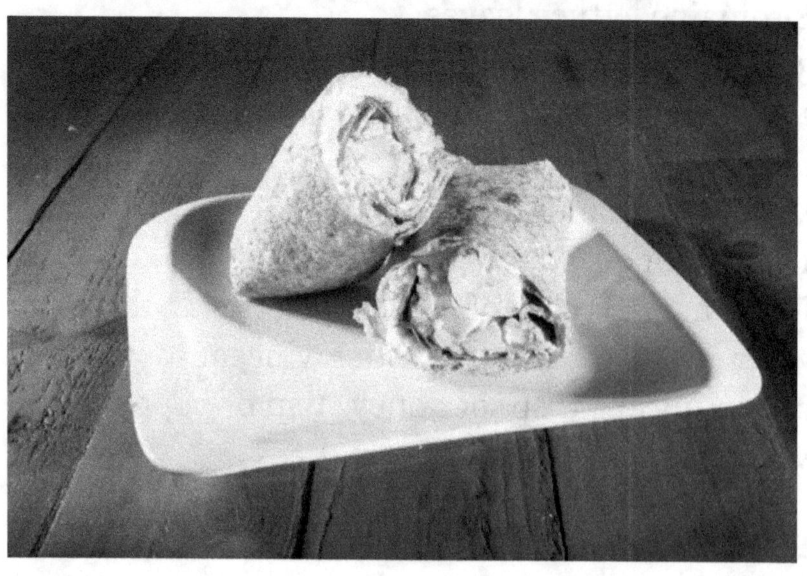

Serving size: 4 servings

Calories: 520 (1 serving)

Preferences: None

Duration: 20 minutes

Ingredients:

- 4 whole wheat tortillas
- 1 avocado (chopped/cubed)
- 1 oz. of chicken (cooked and shredded)
- 1 cup of mozzarella cheese (grated)
- ¼ cup of salsa
- ¼ cup of Greek yogurt
- 1 tbsp. of thyme
- 1 tsp of paprika

Directions:

1. Plate the tortillas and assemble the ingredients.
2. In a bowl, mix the salsa, Greek yogurt, thyme, and paprika.
3. Spread the salsa mixture onto each tortilla.
4. Add chicken, chopped avocado, and mozzarella on top.
5. Wrap the tortillas firmly and slice it in half.
6. Store in airtight containers in the refrigerator for up to three days.

#3 Steak Cobb Salad

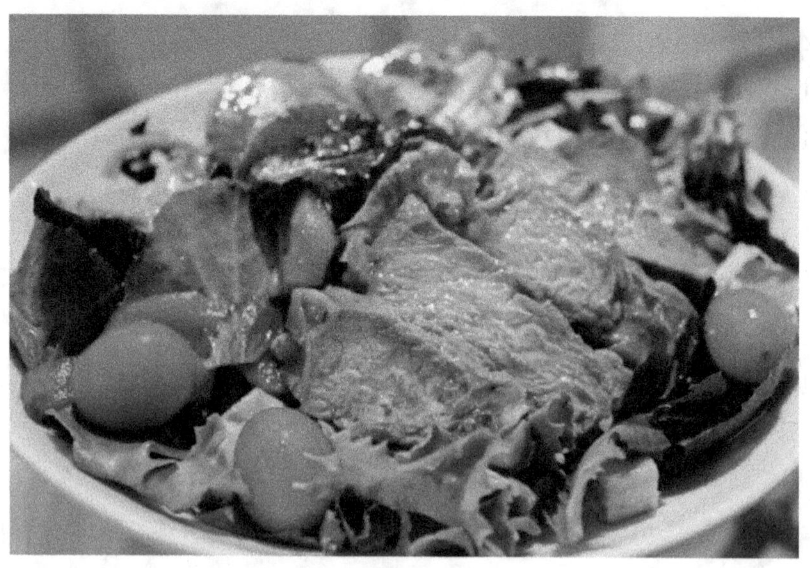

Serving size: 4 servings

Calories: 520 (1 serving)

Preferences: None

Duration: 30 minutes

Ingredients:

- 1 oz. of steak (lean cut)
- 6 eggs (large)
- 6 cups of baby spinach (washed)
- 1 cup of pecan nuts
- 1 cup of rosa tomatoes (sliced)

- ½ cup of feta cheese (cubed)
- 2 tbsps. of butter
- 1 tbsps. of olive oil
- ½ tsp of black pepper
- 1 tsp of Kosher salt

Directions:

1. Melt the butter over medium heat in a large pan.
2. Season the steak with olive oil, salt, and black pepper on both sides, and then add it to the pan. Cook the steak on both sides for 3 to 4 minutes. Cook until it has reached the desired cooking texture (medium-rare).
3. Allow the steak to cool down before cutting it into cubed pieces.
4. Place the eggs in a medium pot, while adding 1 inch of water to the pan.
5. Allow the eggs to come to a boil, and cook it for another minute.
6. Cover the pot with a lid for 8 minutes. Drain the eggs, and allow them to cool before peeling the boiled eggs and cutting them up in quarters.
7. In four separate containers, assemble the salad and divide all the ingredients evenly.
8. Place the baby spinach at the bottom of the container, and top it with a row of steak, tomatoes, eggs, pecan nuts, and feta.
9. Store in airtight containers in the refrigerator for up to three days.

#4 Vegetable Nourish Jars

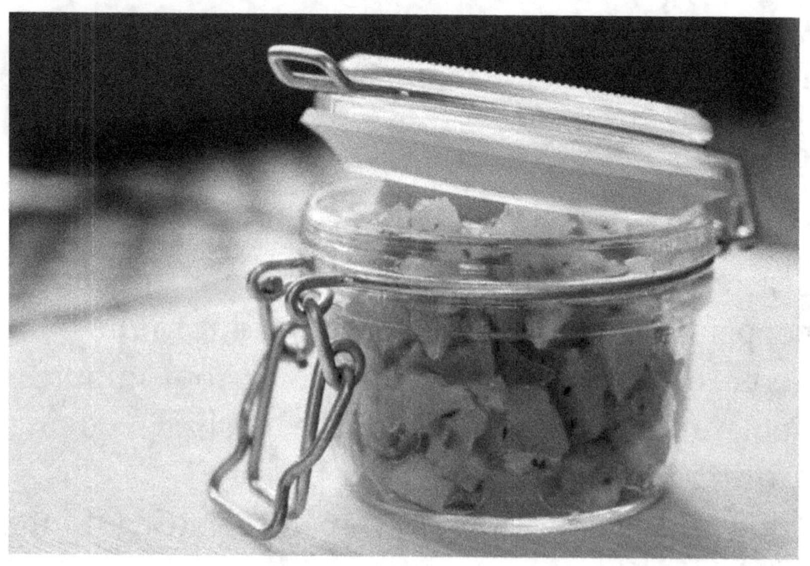

Serving size: 4 servings

Calories: 240 (1 serving)

Preferences: Gluten-free, dairy-free, vegetarian, vegan

Duration: 30 minutes

Ingredients:

- 1 sweet potato (large and cubed)
- 2 cups of baby carrots
- 1 cup of edamame
- 1 cup of cabbage (purple and chopped)
- 1 red bell pepper (diced)
- 1 lime (juice)

- 1 tbsp. of garlic (minced)
- 1 tbsps. of soy sauce (low-sodium)
- 2 tbsp. of olive oil
- ¼ tsp of ginger powder
- ¼ tsp of garlic powder
- ¼ tsp of orange zest
- ½ tsp of black pepper

Directions:

1. Preheat the oven to 400 degrees Fahrenheit, and place the sweet potato and carrots on an oven baking sheet.
2. Drizzle the vegetables, with 1tbsp olive oil, and season it with salt and pepper.
3. Add the minced garlic to the vegetables and roast for 25 minutes.
4. Add the cabbage, red bell pepper, and edamame in a bowl.
5. Mix the lime juice, 1 tbsp. of olive oil, soy sauce, garlic, ginger, and orange zest in a separate bowl.
6. Place the cabbage mixture at the bottom of four medium/large mason jars.
7. Remove the sweet potato and carrots from the oven and place it on top of the cabbage mixture. Drizzle the seasoning on top, and sprinkle with added black pepper.
8. Close the mason jars with lids, and store them in the refrigerator for two to four days.

#5 Mexican Pasta Salad

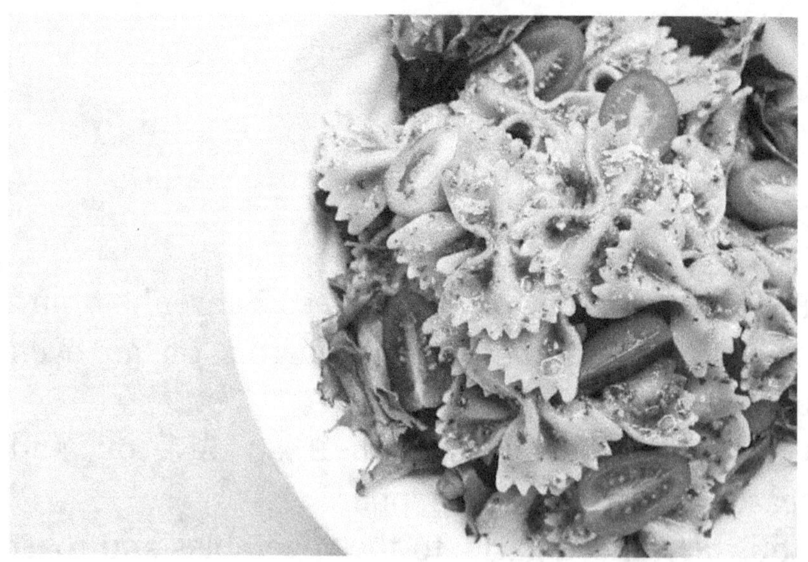

Serving size: 4 servings

Calories: 590 (1 serving)

Preferences: Gluten-free, dairy-free, sugarless

Duration: 30 minutes

Ingredients:

- 10 oz. of pasta (gluten-free)
- 5 strips of lean turkey
- ½ cup of salsa
- ½ cup of cashews (soaked in water for 4+ hours)
- ½ cup of cashew milk
- ½ cup of black beans

- 2 garlic cloves (minced)
- 2 tbsps. of olive oil
- ½ cup of corn
- 1 red bell pepper (diced)
- ½ tsp of chili flakes
- ½ tsp of cumin
- ½ tsp of black pepper

Directions:

1. Cook the pasta for 6-8 minutes in a pot ¾ filled with water over high heat.
2. Drain the pasta, rinse with cold water, and set aside.
3. In a medium-large pan, add olive oil, and cook the turkey until cooked.
4. Once the turkey has cooled down, cut or tear it into small pieces.
5. Add the cashews, cashew milk, salsa, garlic, chili flakes, cumin, and black pepper to a blender. Blend until you've reached a smooth consistency.
6. In four separate containers, divide the pasta, black beans, corn, and bell pepper. Mix all the ingredients, and add the seasoning on top.
7. Store the pasta salad in an airtight container in the refrigerator for up to four days.

#6 Protein Lettuce Wraps

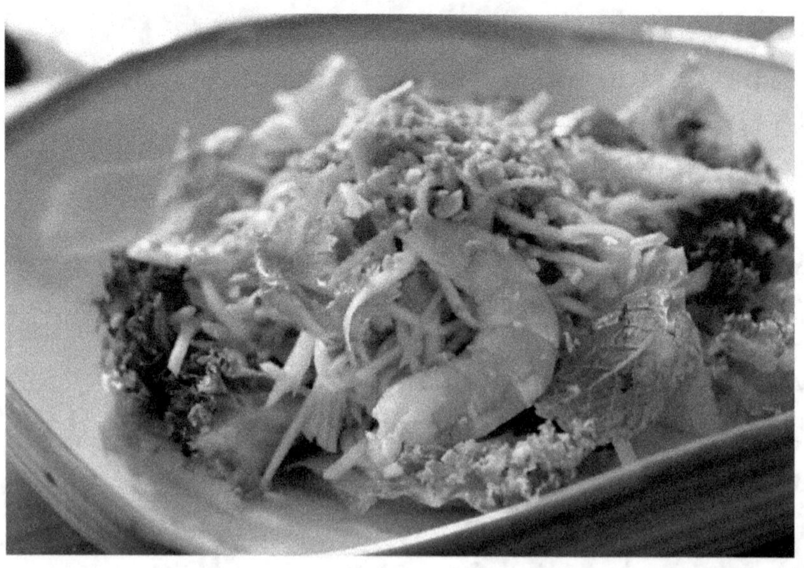

Serving size: 4 servings

Calories: 100 (1 serving)

Preference: Gluten-free, sugarless

Duration: 30 minutes

Ingredients:

- 8 butter lettuce leaves (large)
- 1 lb. shrimp (peeled and deveined)
- ½ cup of cherry tomatoes (sliced)
- 1 tbsp. extra-virgin olive oil
- ½ cup of Greek yogurt
- 1 tsp of dijon mustard
- ½ lemon (juice)
- Kosher salt
- ½ tsp of black pepper

Directions:

1. Preheat oven to 400°F. On a large baking sheet, toss shrimp with oil and season with salt and pepper. Bake until shrimp are completely opaque, 5 to 7 minutes.
2. Mix Greek yogurt, lemon juice, dijon mustard, and black pepper in a bowl.
3. Once mixed, add the shrimps. Mix well.
4. Plate lettuce cups, two per plate, and add 2-3 tablespoons of the shrimp's mixture to it. Add extra black pepper on top. Alternatively, store the lettuce leaves separately from the shrimp's mixture in the refrigerator for up to three days.

#7 French Sandwiches

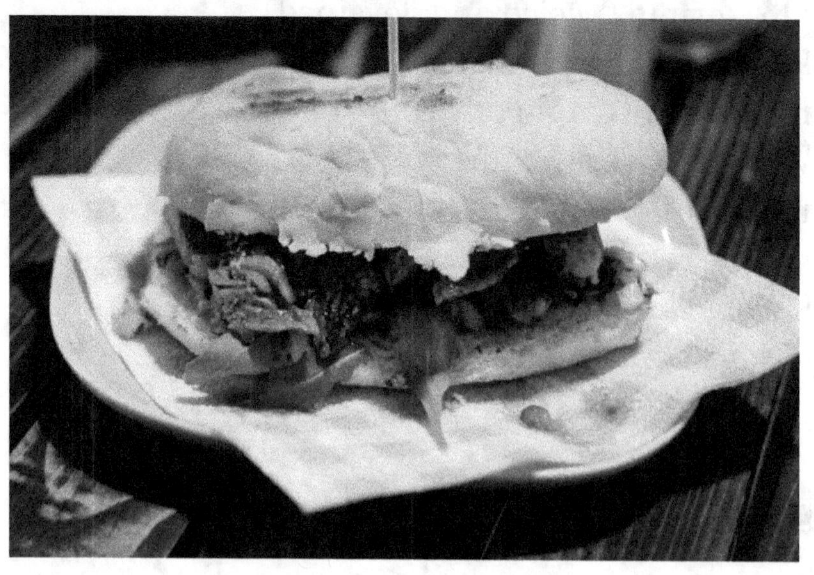

Serving size: 4 servings

Calories: 370 (1 serving)

Preference: Sugarless

Duration: 30 minutes

Ingredients:

- 4 Hawaiian rolls
- 1 lb. of deli-roasted beef (lean)
- 4 slices of mozzarella cheese
- ½ cup of onions (diced and fried)
- Seasoning: 2 tbsps. of butter, ¼ tsp of Worcestershire sauce, ½ tsp of sesame seeds, ¼ tsp of minced garlic, ¼ cup of onion powder, and ¼ cup of Kosher salt.

Directions:

1. Preheat the oven to 350 degrees Fahrenheit.
2. Add slightly melted butter to the bottom of a baking dish.
3. Place the bottom of the Hawaiian rolls in the baking dish, and add deli-roasted beef, fried onions, and 1 slice of cheese on each roll.
4. Mix the seasoning ingredients in a small bowl until well combined.
5. Add the seasoning on top of the other ingredients on the rolls.
6. Cover the rolls with the top part and bake the sandwiches for at least 15 minutes.
7. Remove the sandwiches from the oven, and cut them in half.
8. Serve the sandwiches immediately, or store it by covering them with foil, and placing them in the refrigerator for up to three days.

#8 Teriyaki Chicken

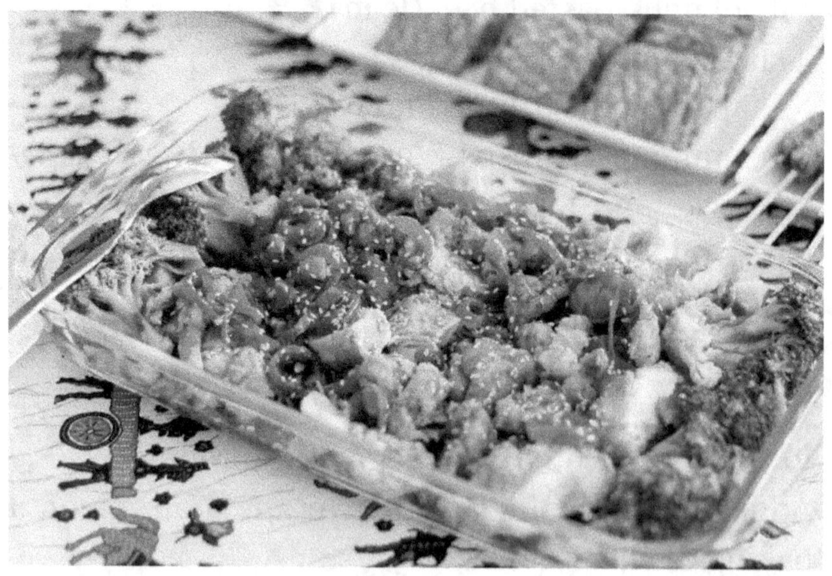

Serving size: 4 servings

Calories: 420 (1 serving)

Preference: Gluten-free, dairy-free

Duration: 30 minutes

Ingredients:

- 3 chicken breasts (halved)
- 3 cups of broccoli
- 1 cup of baby carrots
- ¼ cup of pineapple (chopped)
- ¼ cup of edamame
- 1 spring onion (small and sliced)

- 1 tsp of sesame oil
- 1 tsp of sesame seeds
- Teriyaki sauce: ⅓ cup soy sauce (low-sodium), 5 tbsps. of rice wine vinegar, 5 tbsps. of honey, 2 tsp of sesame oil, 2 garlic cloves (minced), 4 tbsps. of water, ¾ tsp of ginger (grated), and ½ tbsp. of cornstarch.

Directions:

1. Preheat the oven to 400 degrees Fahrenheit and line a sheet pan with parchment paper.
2. Mix all the ingredients of the teriyaki sauce in a bowl.
3. Season the chicken with black pepper, and 2 tsp of teriyaki sauce on both sides of each half. Keep the remaining teriyaki for later.
4. Place the chicken in the middle of the baking sheet, and arrange all of the vegetables around it. Season the chicken and vegetables with more black pepper and a 1 tsp of sesame oil. Place the baking sheet in the oven and cook it for 20 minutes.
5. Remove the pan from the oven and slice the chicken into smaller strips, covering it with the remaining teriyaki sauce.
6. Serve the chicken and vegetables with thin slices of spring onion and sesame seeds on top.
7. Store the chicken and vegetables in airtight containers in the refrigerator for up to four days.

#9 Salmon Salad

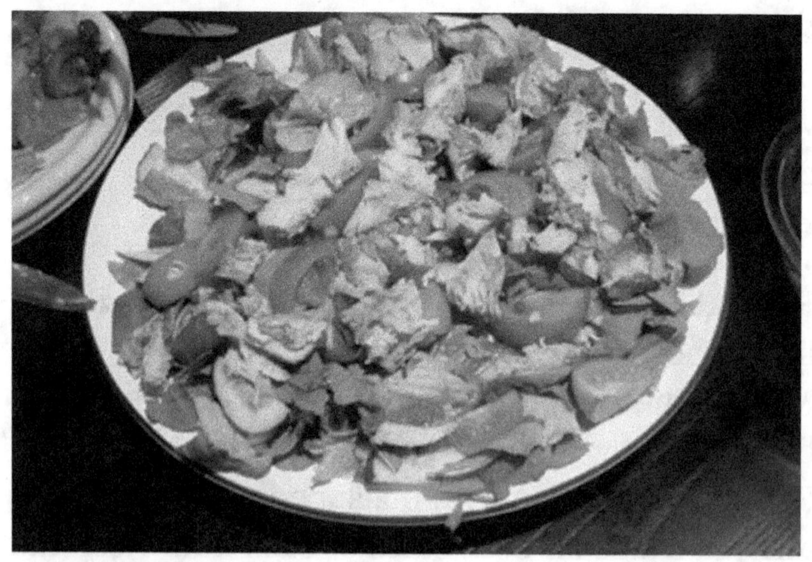

Serving size: 4 servings

Calories: 350 (1 serving)

Preference: Gluten-free, dairy-free, sugarless

Duration: 25 minutes

Ingredients:

- 2 6-oz salmon fillets
- 4 cups of lettuce (chopped)
- 1 cup of cucumber (sliced)
- 1 cup of cherry tomatoes (halved)
- 2 avocado (sliced)
- 2 eggs (boiled)

- 2 tbsp. of olive oil
- 2 tbsp. of lemon juice
- ½ tsp of black pepper
- ½ tsp of garlic powder
- ¼ cup of pickled onions
- ¼ cup of fresh parsley
- Vinaigrette: 3 tbsps. of apple cider vinegar, 1 tbsp. of tahini, 3 tbsps. of olive oil, ½ tsp of garlic powder, ½ tsp of Himalayan salt, and 1 tsp of lemon juice.

Directions:

1. Ensure the salmon is dry on both sides. Then, season it with lemon juice, olive oil, black pepper, and garlic powder.
2. Grill the salmon over medium heat for 5 minutes on both sides, ensuring the fish is cooked on both sides. Flake the cooked salmon into smaller pieces.
3. Mix all of the ingredients for the vinaigrette and drizzle 1 tsp over the avocado.
4. In four separate containers, arrange the lettuce, salmon, eggs, cucumbers, tomatoes, onions, and avocado.
5. Top the salmon salads with fresh parsley, and cover it with airtight lids. Refrigerate for up to three days.

#10 Cauliflower Casserole with Mushrooms and Cheese

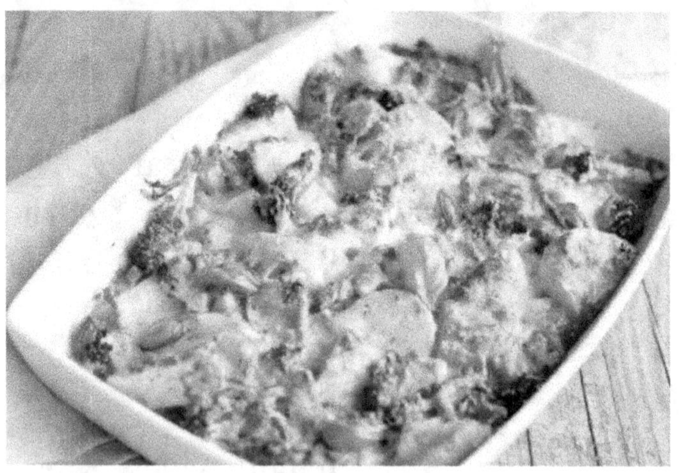

Serving size: 4 servings
Calories: 380 (1 serving)
Preference: Gluten-free, dairy-free, sugarless
Duration: 30 minutes

Ingredients:

- 1 lb. brown mushrooms, chopped
- 3 cups of cauliflower florets
- ½ cup of water
- 1 onion, finely chopped
- 8 oz. of macaroni (gluten-free)
- 1 tbsp. of olive oil
- ½ tsp of garlic powder
- ¼ tsp of black pepper
- ¼ tsp of Himalayan salt
- Sauce: 3 cups of cashew milk, 3 tbsp. of flour (all-purpose), and 8 oz. of cheddar cheese.

<u>*Directions:*</u>

1. Preheat the oven to 375 degrees Fahrenheit. Prepare a casserole dish by spraying it with cooking spray. Set it aside.
2. Chop the cauliflower florets into smaller pieces and place them in the casserole dish.
3. Add olive oil to a pan and saute mushrooms over medium heat. Stir mushrooms once every minute until browned. Add onion and cook for another 5 minutes. Mix in garlic and cook for another minute, then remove from heat, and place them into the casserole dish.
4. Heat 3 cups of cashew milk over medium heat and stir the milk frequently. Add flour to the milk a tbsp. at a time, and continue stirring it to ensure it doesn't burn.
5. Once you've reached a thick texture, switch the heat to low, and add the cheddar cheese. Continue stirring the sauce. Add a pinch of salt, black pepper, and garlic powder to the sauce. Pour the sauce over the mushrooms and cauliflower. Then, add the water on top, ensuring everything is combined well. Bake the mushrooms and vegetables for 20 minutes in the oven.
6. Removing the casserole dish from the oven, stir in the noodles, mixing all the ingredients, and cooking it for five more minutes.
7. Divide the mac and cheese into four containers and refrigerate it up to four days.

Dinner Recipes

#1 Couscous Salad

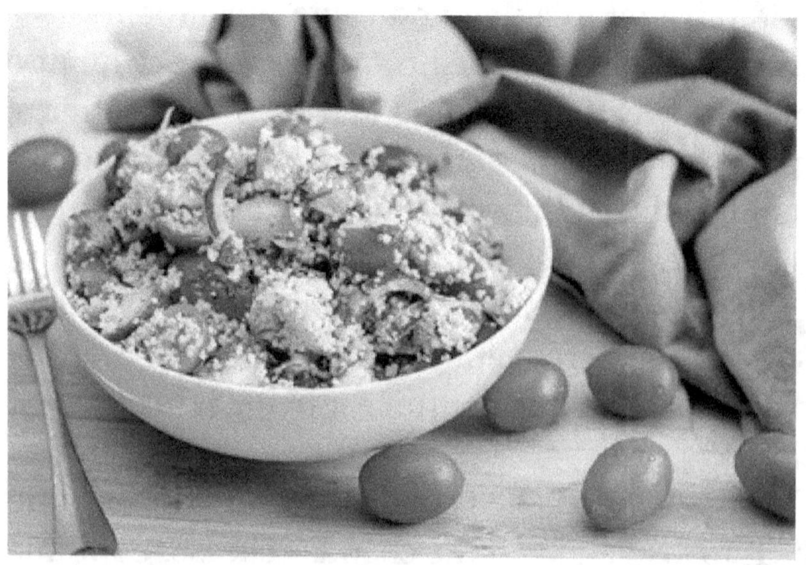

Serving size: 4 servings

Calories: 470 (1 serving)

Preference: Sugarless

Duration: 25 minutes

Ingredients:

- 15 oz. of chickpeas (1 can)
- 5 oz. mozzarella cheese (grated)
- 5 oz. of salami (chopped)

- 5 oz. of olives (halved)
- 2 4.7-oz of Couscous (packages)
- 1 green bell pepper (chopped)
- 2 cups of cherry tomatoes
- ¾ cup of basil
- Dressing: ⅓ cup of red wine vinegar, ¾ cup of olive oil, 1 tbsp. of dijon mustard, 1 tsp of garlic (minced), 1 tsp of honey, ½ tsp of basil, ½ tsp of oregano, ½ tsp of thyme, and ¼ tsp of red chili flakes.

Directions:

1. Prepare the couscous according to the package instructions.
2. While the couscous is busy cooking in a pan, prepare the salad.
3. Add the chickpeas, salami, mozzarella, bell pepper, tomatoes, olives, and basil in a bowl, and mix everything.
4. Add the dressing to a jar and shake it until the ingredients are combined. Add extra salt and pepper if preferred.
5. In four mason jars, divide the couscous evenly. Place half of a couscous serving at the bottom of each jar, and then top it with the salad mixture. Add the remaining serving half on top, and stir everything together in the jars.
6. Refrigerate the couscous mason jars for up to three days.

#2 Sesame Noodles

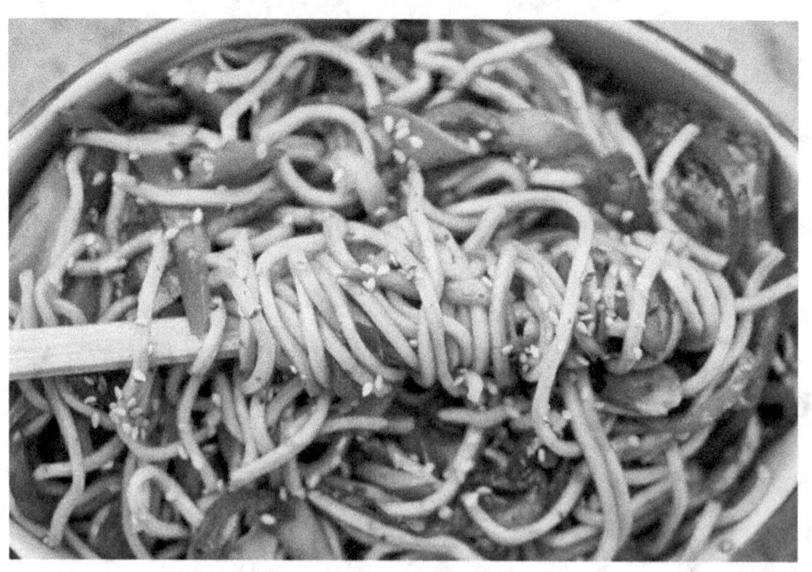

Serving size: 4 servings

Calories: 450 (1 serving)

Preference: Dairy-free, sugarless

Duration: 15 minutes

Ingredients:

- 6 oz. of stir fry noodles (whole wheat)
- 2 cucumbers
- 2 cups of edamame (cooked)
- 1 lb. chicken breast (cooked and chopped)
- 1 tsp of sesame seeds
- Sesame sauce: ¼ cup of tahini, ¼ cup of hot water, 2 tbsps. of soy sauce, 1 tbsp. of rice vinegar, 1 tbsp. of sesame oil, 1 tsp of brown sugar, and 1 clove of garlic.

Directions:

1. Whisk the sesame sauce's ingredients together. Ensure the sauce is a smooth consistency.
2. For the noodles, cook it according to package instructions. Once done, rinse it in cold water and add ½ of the sesame sauce on top. Mix well.
3. Divide the noodles, cooked edamame, chicken, and cucumber into four containers. Sprinkle sesame seeds on top, and store it in the refrigerator for up to four days. Serve cold.

#3 Cauliflower Tacos

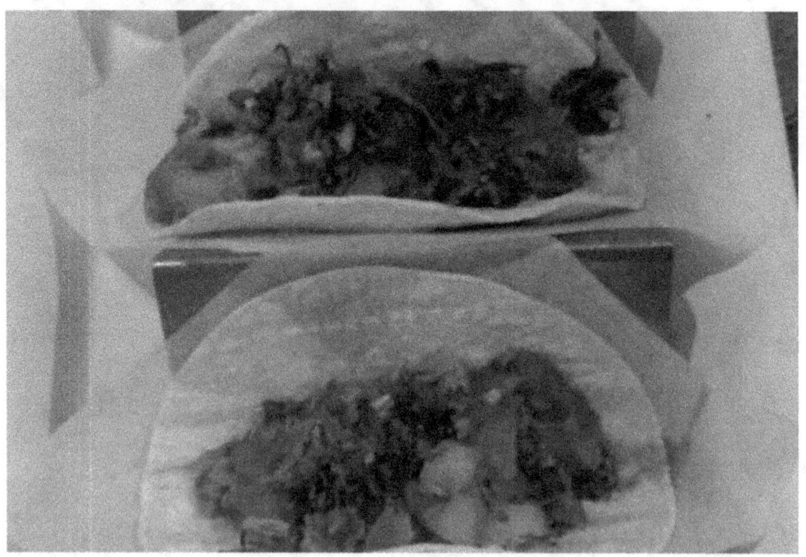

Serving size: 4 servings Cauliflower Tacos

Calories: 460 (1 serving)

Preference: Dairy-free, vegetarian, vegan, sugarless

Duration: 30 minutes

Ingredients:

- 2 small cauliflower heads (chopped)
- 4 tbsps. of avocado oil
- 3 tsp of cumin
- 2 tsp of chili flakes
- 1 tsp of basil
- 1 tsp of Kosher salt
- Sauce: 4 garlic cloves, ¼ cup of almonds (raw), one 15-oz can of cherry tomatoes

- 2 tbsps. of olive oil
- 1 medium lime (juice)
- Seasoning: ¼ tsp of Kosher salt, 1 tbsp. of maple syrup, ½ tsp of cilantro, ½ tsp of paprika, and 2 whole chipotle peppers
- Serving: 12 corn tortillas (plantain), and ¼ cup of red cabbage (sliced), lime juice (wedges), and 1 avocado (sliced)

Directions:

1. Preheat the oven to 400 degrees Fahrenheit.
2. Add the cauliflower onto 2 baking sheets avocado oil on top. Season the cauliflower with cumin, chili flakes, basil, and salt. Roast the cauliflower on the bottom rack of the oven for 20 minutes.
3. On a separate baking sheet, toast the almonds with the garlic cloves (peeled) for 10 minutes. Remove and set it aside.
4. Once the cauliflower is finished roasting, add the seasoning ingredients to a blender and blend it on high speed until it reaches a smooth consistency.
5. Serve the tacos hot. Place the cauliflower florets inside and drizzle the seasoning on top.
6. Fold the tortillas into tacos, and add red cabbage, a drizzle of lime juice, and avocado on top if preferred.
7. Store the cauliflower tacos in an airtight container for up to three das.

#4 Spicy Quinoa Jars (Vegetarian)

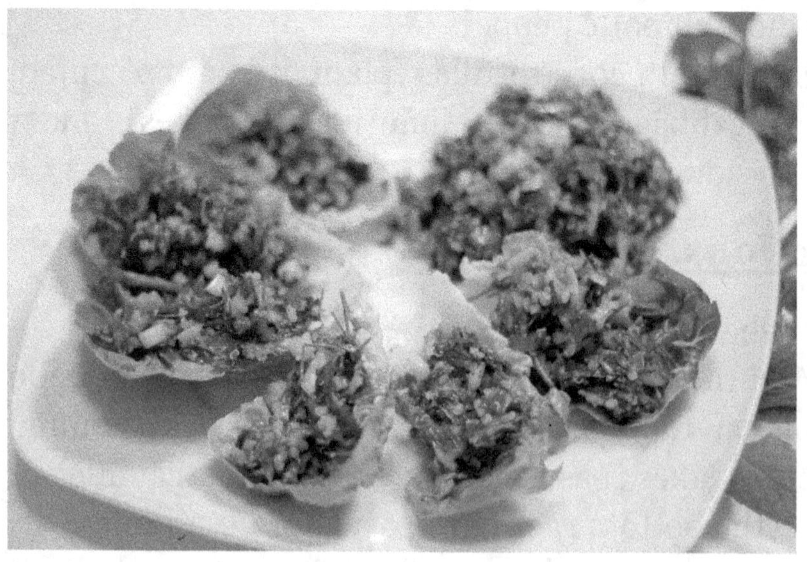

Serving size: 4 servings

Calories: 540 (1 serving)

Preference: Gluten-free, dairy-free, vegetarian, vegan, sugarless

Duration: 15 minutes

Ingredients:

- 3 cups of quinoa (cooked)
- 3 avocados (halved)
- 1 cup of corn
- 2 romaine lettuce heads (chopped)
- 15 oz. of black beans
- ½ cup of salsa
- ½ cup of cilantro
- 1 tsp of coriander
- 1 lime (juice)

Directions:

1. In a large bowl, mix the quinoa, corn, beans, cilantro, lime juice, and spices. Combine the ingredients well.

2. Add 2 cups of romaine lettuce at the bottom of four mason jars. Then, add 1-½ cups of the quinoa mixture with 1 tbsp. of salsa and ½ avocado on top.

3. Add lime juice and cilantro on top.

4. Seal the mason jars, and refrigerate them for up to five days.

#5 Turkey Breasts and Vegetables

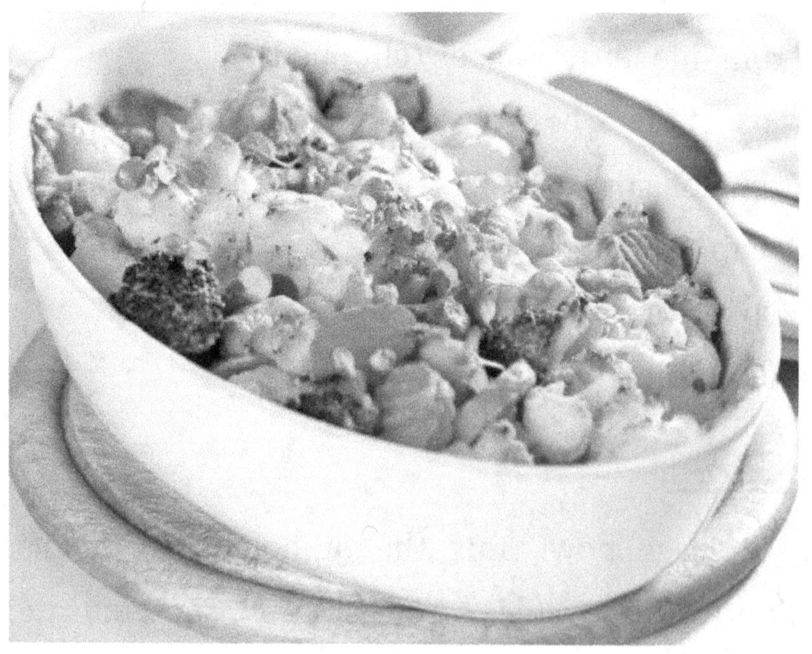

Serving size: 4 servings

Calories: 460 (1 serving)

Preference: Sugarless

Duration: 30 minutes

Ingredients:

- 16 oz. of turkey breasts (lean and chopped)
- 2 cups of potatoes (peeled, washed, and chopped)
- 2 cups of baby carrots

- 2-⅓ cups of baby marrow (chopped)
- 2 cups of red bell peppers (chopped)
- 1-½ cup of broccoli florets
- ⅓ cup of feta cheese (crumbled)
- Seasoning: ½ tbsp. of oregano, ½ tbsp. of basil, ½ tbsp. of parsley, ½ tbsp. of garlic powder, ½ tsp of thyme, ⅛ tp of red pepper flakes, 4-½ tbsps. of olive oil

Directions:

1. Preheat the oven to 400 degrees Fahrenheit and line a sheet pan with parchment paper. Set it aside.
2. Add the prepped vegetables and chopped turkey breasts to the sheet pan.
3. Prepare the seasoning by mixing the ingredients in a bowl. Drizzle the seasoning on top of the turkey breasts and vegetables.
4. Place the sheet pan in the oven. Allow it to cook for 15 minutes. Remove the sheet and toss the turkey breasts and vegetables around before returning it to the oven. Allow it to cook for 10 more minutes.
5. Add the feta cheese on top once done and serve it either on its own or with whole grain.
6. Divide the turkey breasts and vegetables evenly between four separate airtight containers and store it in the refrigerator for up to three days.

#6 Buffalo Tofu Jars

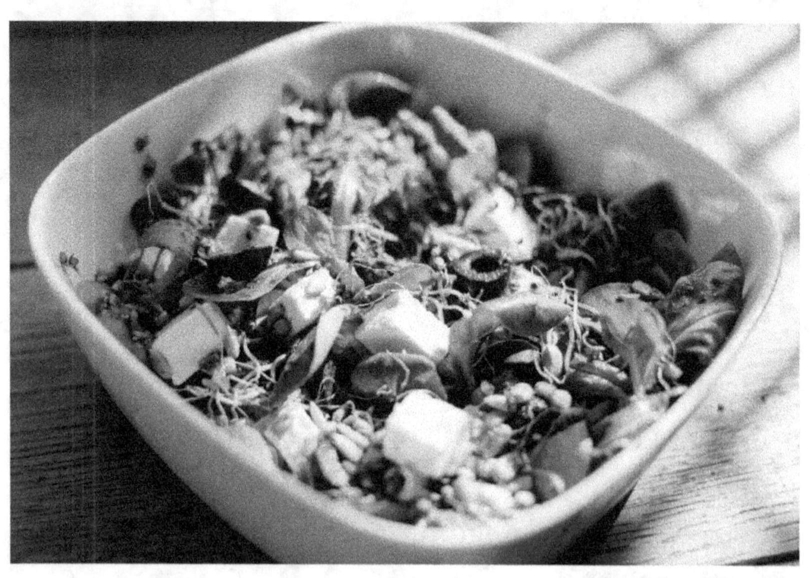

Serving size: 4 servings

Calories: 90 (1 serving)

Preference: Gluten-free, dairy-free, vegetarian, vegan, sugarless

Duration: 15 minutes

Ingredients:

- 8 cups of romaine lettuce (shredded)
- 2 cups of tofu (firm and cubed)
- 2 cups of celery (chopped)
- 2 cups of carrots (shredded)
- 2 cups of rosa tomatoes (chopped)
- ½ cup of buffalo sauce (vegan)
- Dressing: 4 tbsps. of tahini, 1 tsp of garlic powder, 1 tsp of Himalayan salt, 2 lemons (juice)

Directions:

1. Mix the buffalo sauce and tofu in a bowl, and set it aside.
2. Mix all of the salad ingredients in a large bowl.
3. Mix the dressing ingredients in a separate bowl and divide it into four portions.
4. To four mason jars, add the salad ingredients with the seasoned tofu on top. Layer the ingredients as preferred.
5. Refrigerate the mason jar containers for up to three days, and serve chilled.

7 Honey Sriracha Meatballs

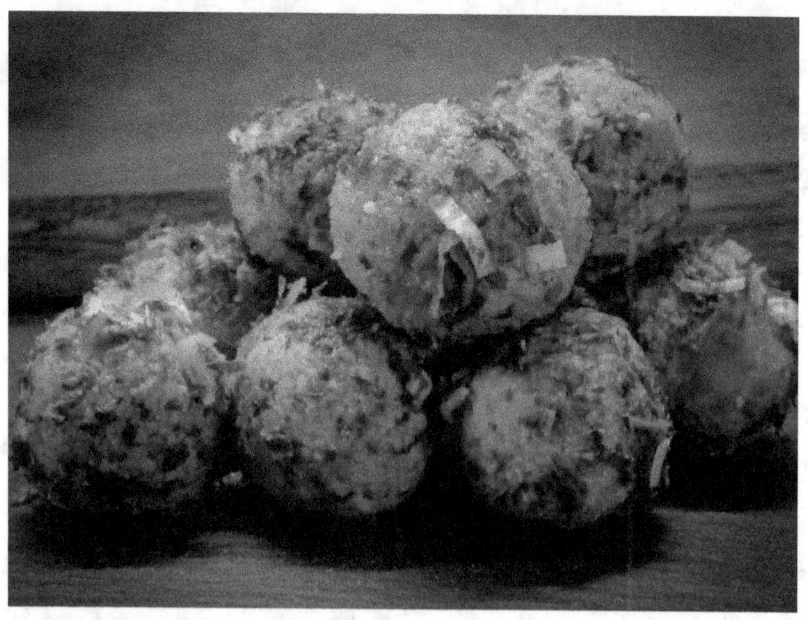

Serving size: 4 servings

Calories: 250 (1 serving)

Preference: Dairy-free, vegetarian

Duration: 30 minutes

Ingredients:

- 1 lb. of turkey (ground)
- 1 egg
- ½ cup of breadcrumbs (whole wheat)
- ⅛ cup of onions (chopped)
- ¼ tsp of garlic powder

- ¼ tsp of black pepper
- Sauce: 1-½ tbsps. of rice vinegar, 1-½ tbsps. of soy sauce, 1-½ tbsps. of honey, 1-½ garlic cloves (minced), ⅛ cup of sriracha, ½ tsp of ginger (grated), and ¼ tsp of sesame oil.

Directions:

1. Preheat the oven to 375 degrees Fahrenheit.
2. Mix the turkey, egg, breadcrumbs, onions, black pepper, and garlic powder in a bowl until everything is well combined.
3. Shape the turkey mixture into 1-½-inch individual meatballs (about 20).
4. Prepare a baking sheet by spraying it with cooking spray, and bake it for 20 minutes.
5. While the meatballs are in the oven, combine the sauce ingredients in a separate bowl and whisk everything together well.
6. Add sauce mixture to a saucepan and allow it to boil over medium heat for 8 minutes while stirring it continuously.
7. Remove the meatballs from the oven and add it to the saucepan, ensuring it is well covered in sauce.
8. Serve the meatballs on top of a serving of brown rice with onions.
9. Place the honey sriracha meatballs in four containers in the refrigerator, and cover it with airtight lids for up to four days.

#8 Red Lentil Dal

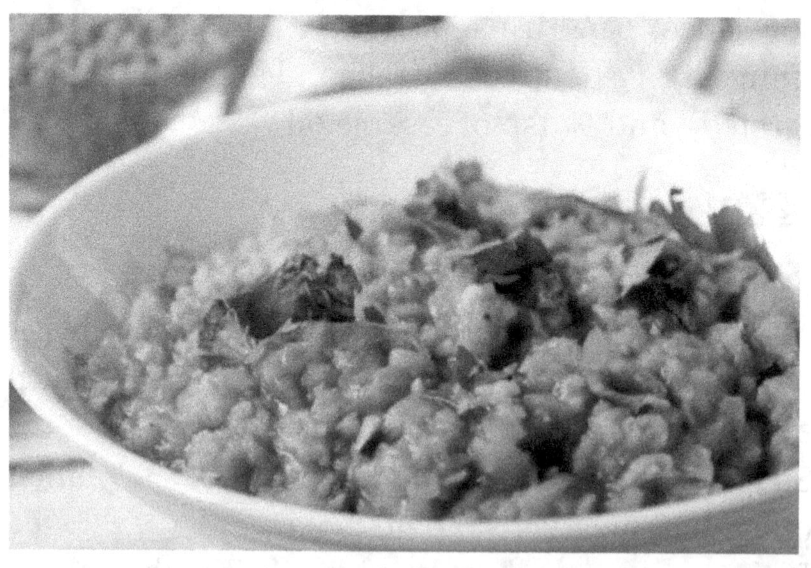

Serving size: 4 servings

Calories: 250 (1 serving)

Preference: Gluten-free, dairy-free, vegetarian, vegan, sugarless

Duration: 15 minutes

Ingredients:

- 2 cups of red lentils (dried)
- 1-½ cup of quinoa (cooked)
- 1 oz of coconut milk (can)
- 1-½ tsp of turmeric
- ½ tsp of cumin
- ½ tsp of ginger
- ½ tsp of curry powder
- ½ tsp of black pepper

Directions:

1. Add the coconut milk and red lentils to a pot over medium heat, and allow it to come to a boil. Then, cook it for 10 minutes.

2. Stir in the turmeric, cumin, curry powder, ginger, and black pepper. Cook for another 5 minutes.

3. In four separate containers, add the quinoa, and top it with the spicy coconut-lentil mixture. Close it with lids, and store it in the refrigerator for up to three days.

#9 Spaghetti Squash Boats

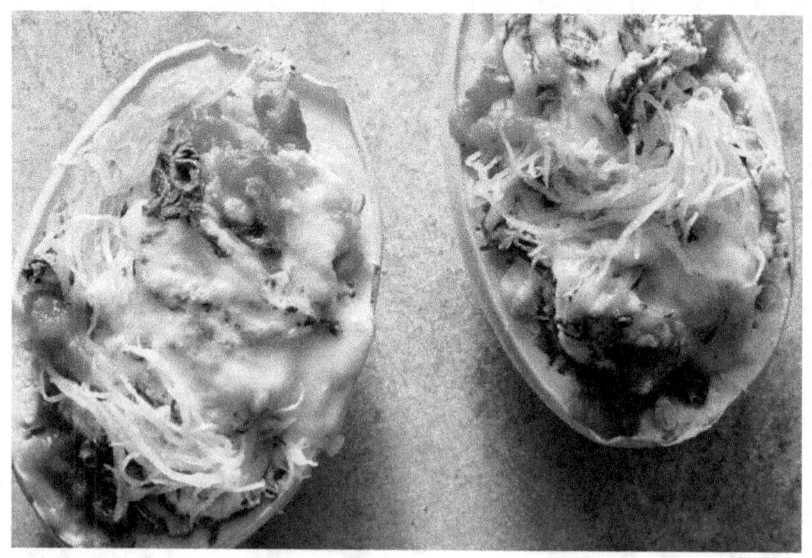

Serving size: 4 servings

Calories: 300 (1 serving)

Preference: Gluten-free, vegetarian

Duration: 30 minutes

Ingredients:

- 2 cans of diced tomatoes
- 2 spaghetti squash (halved)
- ½ cup of hummus
- ½ cup of red lentils
- ¼ cup of nutritional yeast

- 1 tbsp. of Italian seasoning
- ½ cup of water
- ½ tsp of salt
- ½ cup of mozzarella cheese (shredded)

Directions:

1. Preheat the oven to 420 degrees Fahrenheit.
2. Take the halved squash and place them face down on a baking dish. Add the water to the baking dish, ensuring it covers at least a ¼ of the squash. Roast the squash for 20 minutes in the oven.
3. In the meantime, add diced tomatoes, red lentils, nutritional yeast, Italian seasoning, salt, and hummus to a saucepan. Stir the ingredients frequently, and add 1 cup of water to the pan. Allow it to boil and then simmer for 10 minutes.
4. Remove the squash from the oven once done. Scoop out all the seeds, and fill the squash with 1 cup of sauce.
5. Place it back in the oven for 2 minutes. Add the cheese on top of the squash while still hot, allowing it to melt.
6. Store the squash in airtight containers for up to three days.

#10 Spicy Chicken with Rice

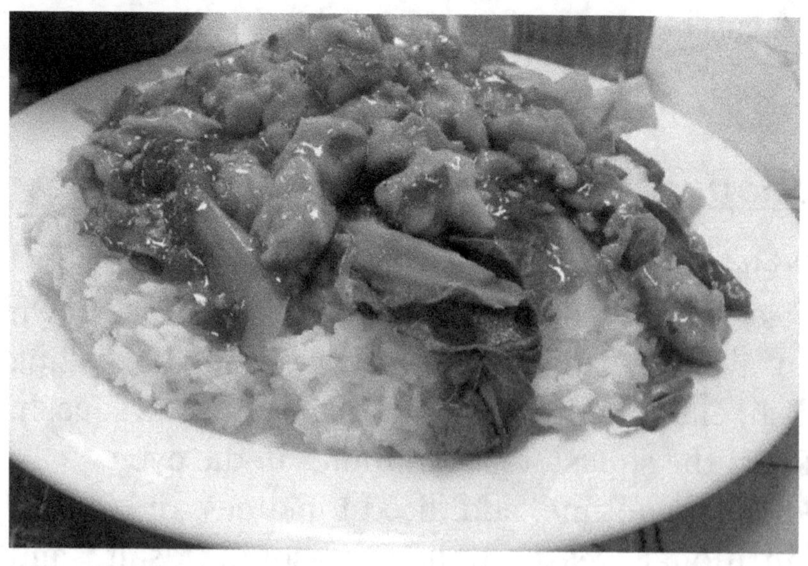

Serving size: 4 servings

Calories: 510 (1 serving)

Preference: Dairy-free

Duration: 10 minutes

Ingredients:

- 1 cup of brown rice
- 1 cup of water
- 14 oz. of salsa
- 1 lb. of chicken breasts
- 1 14 oz. of black beans
- ½ tsp of salt
- ½ tsp of chili powder
- ½ tsp of cayenne pepper
- ½ tsp of garlic powder
- 1 tbsp. of cilantro (fresh)

Directions:

1. Place the rice tomatoes, salt, oil, and water into one pot. Stir the ingredients to combine.
2. Place the chicken in the pot with the spices and salt. Switch the heat to high heat, and cook the ingredients for 8 minutes.
3. Once done, turn down the heat to low.
4. Remove the chicken from the pot, and set it aside.
5. Mix the black beans into the pot, and allow it to cook for 2 minutes.
6. Place the cooked ingredients in four separate containers.
7. Add fresh cilantro, and drizzle some of the remaining sauce in the pot on top.
8. Store it in the refrigerator in airtight containers for up to three days.

Snack Recipes

#1 Avocado Chips

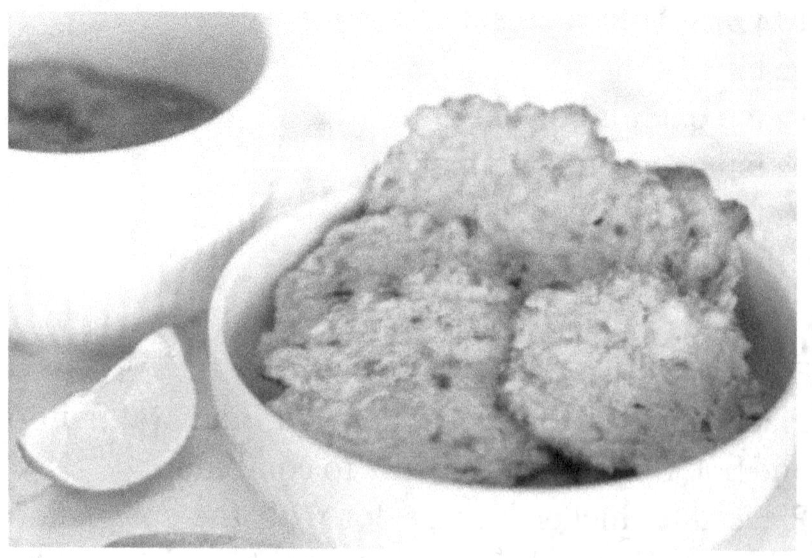

Serving size: 4 servings

Calories: 100 (1 serving)

Preference: Gluten-free, vegetarian, vegan, sugarless

Duration: 30 minutes

Ingredients:

- 1 avocado (large)
- ¾ cup of mozzarella cheese (grated)
- 1 tsp of lemon juice
- ½ tsp of Italian seasoning
- ½ tsp of black pepper
- ½ tsp of salt

Directions:

1. Preheat the oven to 325 degrees Fahrenheit and line two baking sheets with parchment paper.
2. Mash the avocado in a medium bowl. Then, add in the lemon juice, salt, black pepper, Italian seasoning, and mozzarella cheese.
3. Scoop a tbsp. of the mixture at a time onto the baking sheet, leaving 3 inches between each dollop of avocado mixture. Flatten each scoop, until it reaches a 3-inch width.
4. Bake the chips for 30 minutes in the oven, and then allow it to cool down.
5. Serve the chips immediately, or divide it into four servings in Ziploc bags. Store at room temperature in the pantry for up to a week.

#2 Chocolate Bark

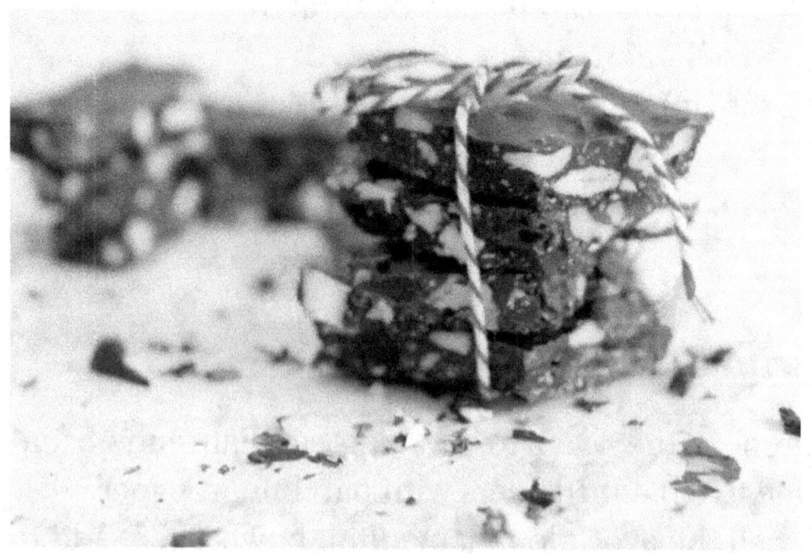

Serving size: 4+ servings

Calories: 250 (1 serving)

Preference: None

Duration: 15 minutes + 1 hour refrigerate

Ingredients:

- 2 bags of dark choc chips (12 oz, melted)
- ½ cup of pretzels (chopped)
- ¼ cup of coconut flakes
- ¼ cup of dried cranberries
- ¼ cup of pistachios
- Sea salt

Directions:

1. Line a baking sheet with parchment paper.
2. Pour ⅓ of the melted chocolate onto the baking sheet. Use a spoon to spread everything until it is layered on the baking sheet.
3. Sprinkle half of the cranberries, coconut, pretzels, and coconut on top.
4. Pour the remaining ⅔ chocolate over the baking sheet. Then sprinkle the remaining ingredients on top.
5. Add sea salt on top.
6. Allow the chocolate bark to set in the refrigerator for 1 hour.
7. Break the bark into pieces once set. Place it in an airtight container until ready to eat as a snack.

#3 Deviled Eggs with Hummus

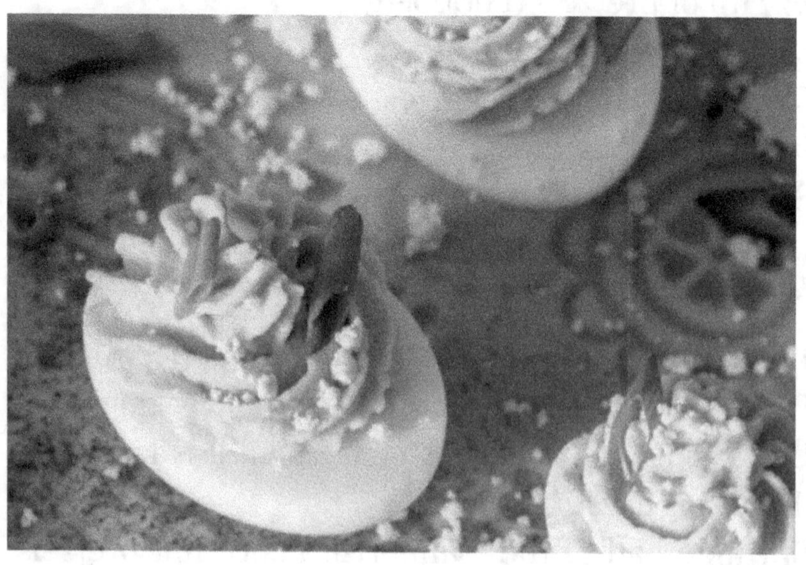

Serving size: 4 servings

Calories: 240 (1 serving)

Preference: Gluten-free, dairy-free, sugarless

Duration: 20 minutes

<u>*Ingredients:*</u>

- 8 eggs
- ½ cup of hummus (smooth)
- ½ tsp of Kosher salt
- ½ tsp of black pepper
- ¼ cup of onion (diced and cooked)

<u>*Directions:*</u>

1. Place the eggs in a pot, covering it with 1 to 2 inches of cold water. Place the pot on the stove, allow to broil, before covering the pot for 10 minutes.
2. Remove the eggs from the pot and place them in cold water.
3. Once the eggs are cold, peel them, slice them in half, remove the yellow part, and place it in a bowl.
4. Mix the yellow part of the egg with hummus, salt, and pepper.
5. Scoop the hummus-egg mixture into the halved white eggs.
6. Place the deviled eggs in an airtight container for up to three days.

#4 Paleo Granola

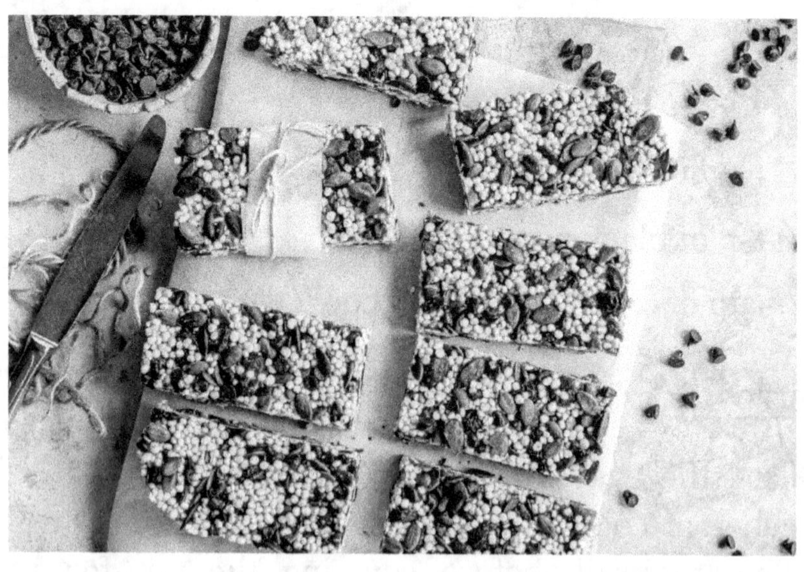

Serving size: 4 servings

Calories: 530 (1 serving)

Preference: Dairy-free, vegetarian

Duration: 30 minutes

Ingredients:

- 1 cup of pecan nuts
- 1 cup of almonds
- 1 cup of cranberries

- ½ cup of coconut flakes
- ½ cup of pumpkin seeds
- ¼ cup of flaxseeds
- ¼ cup of sunflower seeds
- 3 tbsps. of coconut oil
- 1 tsp of cinnamon
- ½ tsp of nutmeg
- ¼ cup of honey
- 1 tsp of vanilla extract

<u>*Directions:*</u>

1. Preheat the oven to 350 degrees Fahrenheit and spray cooking spray on a baking sheet.
2. Mix the nuts, seeds, and spices in a bowl.
3. In a separate bowl, mix the vanilla, honey, and coconut oil.
4. Pour the wet mixture over the nut-seed mixture, and spread the granola on the baking sheet evenly.
5. Bake the granola for 20 minutes.
6. Once done, remove from the oven and allow it to cool down.
7. Store the granola in an airtight jar or divide it into Ziploc bags. Store it at room temperature for up to three weeks.

#5 Protein Balls

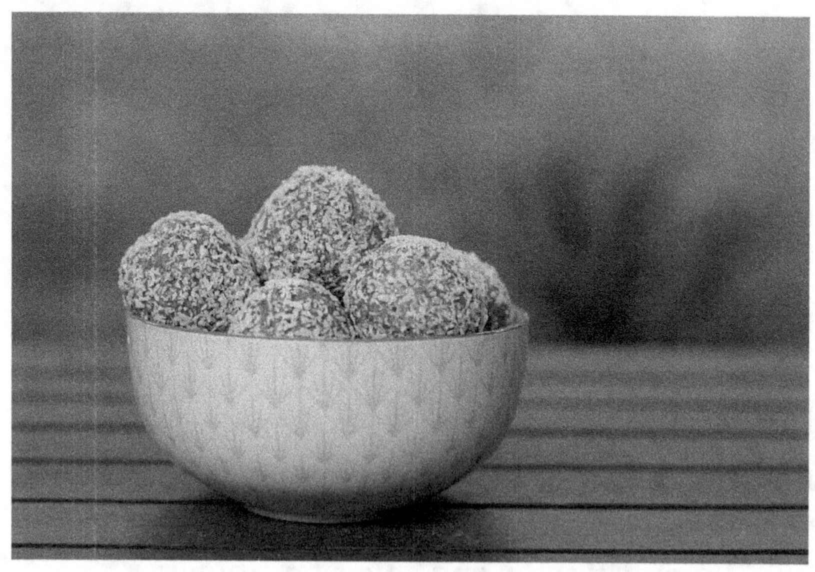

Serving size: 4+ servings

Calories: 360 (1 serving)

Preference: Vegetarian

Duration: 30 minutes

Ingredients:

- ½ cup of shredded coconut
- ¼ cup of rolled oats
- ¼ cup of chocolate chips
- ¼ cup of honey
- ¾ cup of natural peanut butter
- 2 tbsps. of chia seeds
- 2 tbsps. of flaxseeds
- 2 tbsps. of nut milk
- ½ tsp of vanilla extract
- ¼ tsp of cinnamon
- ¼ tsp of Himalayan salt

Directions:

1. Line a baking sheet with parchment paper.
2. Mix the rolled oats, coconut, chia seeds, flaxseeds, chocolate chips, salt, and cinnamon in a bowl until everything is well combined. Then, add the peanut butter, vanilla extract, and honey. Ensure the mixture is slightly crumbly, and not too dry, otherwise stir in the milk.
3. Roll the protein mixture into balls, about 3 inches wide, and place them on a baking sheet 1 to 2 inches apart.
4. Refrigerate the mixture for 30 minutes before serving. Or, place it into airtight containers, and serve on the go as a snack.

#6 Chocolate-Dipped Clementines

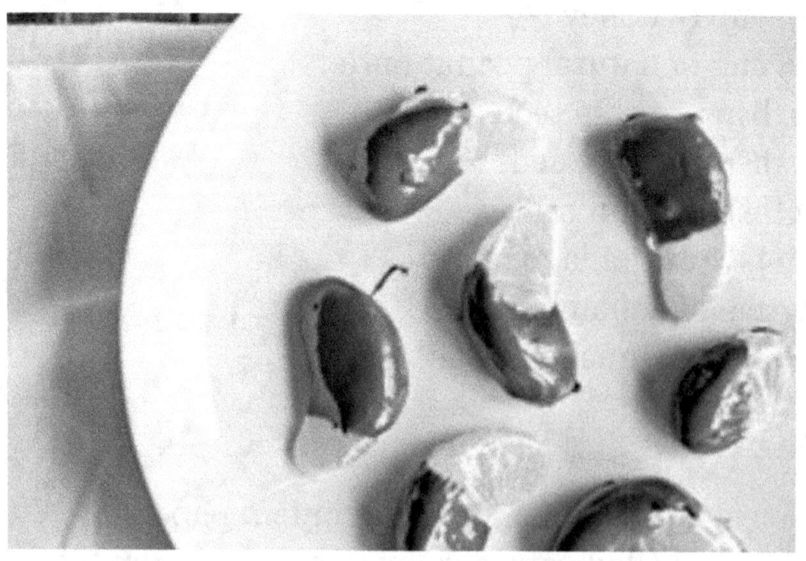

Serving size: 4+ servings

Calories: 120 (1 serving)

Preference: Gluten-free, vegetarian

Duration: 20 minutes

<u>*Ingredients:*</u>

- 5 clementine oranges (peeled and divided)
- ¼ cup of chocolate chips (melted)
- 1 tsp of coconut oil
- ½ tsp of sea salt

<u>*Directions:*</u>

1. Stir the coconut oil and melted chocolate together.

2. Dip the clementine segments in the melted chocolate mixture.

3. Transfer the clementine segments to a baking sheet lined with parchment paper.

4. Add sea salt on top, and refrigerate it for 20 minutes.

5. Serve immediately, or place in a container for up to three days.

#7 Sweet and Salty Nuts

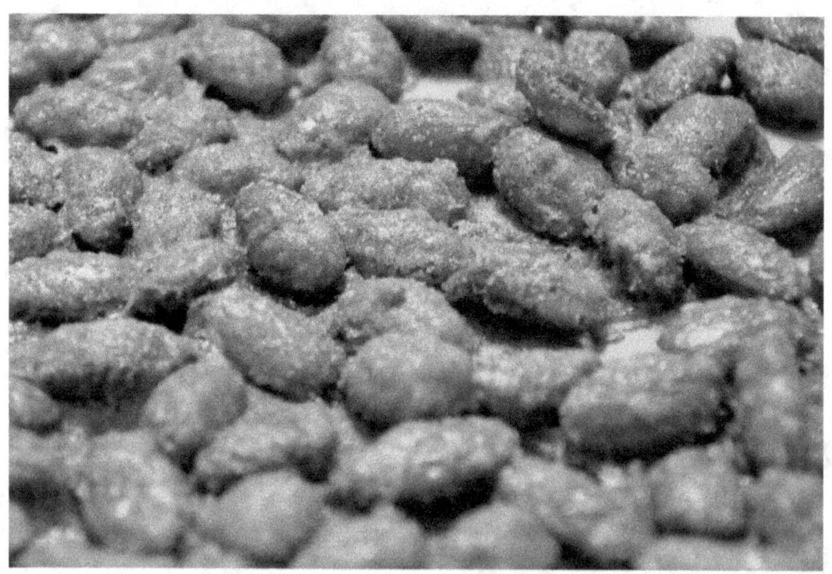

Serving size: 4 servings

Calories: 300 (1 serving)

Preference: Gluten-free, dairy-free, vegetarian

Duration: 15 minutes

Ingredients:

- 3 cups of raw almonds
- 1 egg white
- ⅓ quinoa
- 2 tbsps. of honey
- ¼ tsp of cayenne pepper
- ¼ tsp of ground ginger
- ½ tsp of Kosher salt

Directions:

1. Preheat the oven to 300 degrees Fahrenheit, and place parchment paper to fit on a baking sheet.
2. Mix the almonds, quinoa, egg white, honey, ginger, and cayenne pepper in a bowl. Add the salt.
3. Pour mixture onto the baking sheet, and bake until the mixture is toasted for 15 minutes.
4. Remove the nuts from the oven, and divide it into four Ziploc bags. Store at room temperature for up to a month.

#8 Wholesome Crackers

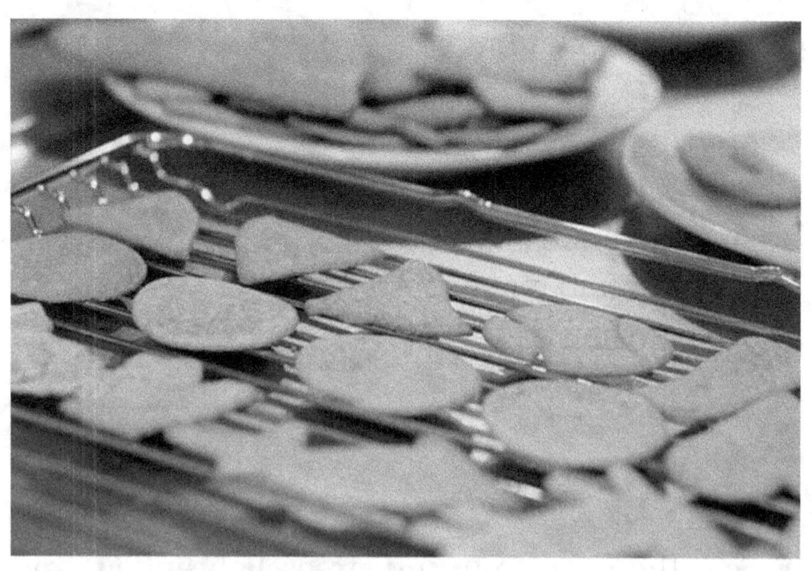

Serving size: 4+ servings

Calories: 330 (1 serving)

Preference: Gluten-free, dairy-free, vegetarian, sugarless

Duration: 20 minutes

Ingredients:

- 3 eggs
- 2-½ cups of almond flour
- ½ cup of coconut flour
- 1 tsp of flaxseed meal (ground)
- ½ tsp of onion powder
- ½ tsp of rosemary (chopped)
- ¼ tsp of Himalayan salt
- 1 tbsp. of olive oil

Directions:

1. Preheat the oven to 325 degrees Fahrenheit and line a baking sheet with parchment paper.
2. Mix the almond flour, coconut flour, flaxseed meal, onion powder, salt, and rosemary in a bowl.
3. Add the oil and eggs to the dry ingredients.
4. Mix the ingredients until you have a dough.
5. Sandwich the dough between two single pieces of parchment paper. Roll the dough ¼ of an inch thick, and cut it into squares. Transfer it to a baking sheet.
6. Bake the crackers for 10 minutes and allow it to cool down before placing it in an airtight container.
7. Store the container in the refrigerator for up to two weeks.

#9 Tortilla Chips with Guacamole

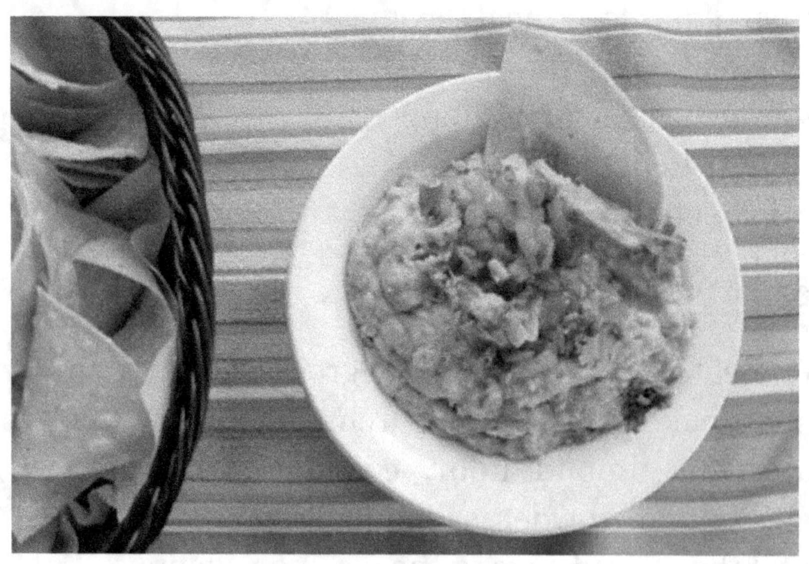

Serving size: 4 servings

Calories: 330 (1 serving)

Preference: Gluten-free, vegetarian, sugarless

Duration: 30 minutes

Ingredients:

- 2 cups of mozzarella (shredded)
- 1 cup of almond flour
- 1 tsp of Himalayan salt
- 1 tsp of garlic powder
- ½ tsp of cayenne pepper
- ½ tsp of black pepper
- 1 cup of guacamole (store-bought)

Directions:

1. Preheat the oven to 350 degrees Fahrenheit and line two baking sheets with parchment paper.
2. Add the mozzarella to a microwaveable bowl and microwave for 1-½ minutes.
3. Add the almond flour, cayenne pepper, salt, garlic powder, and black pepper to the cheese to create a dough.
4. Knead the dough with your hands until it is smooth.
5. Place the dough between 2 sheets of parchment paper. Roll out the dough, and cut large strips of dough into ⅛-inch thick rectangles.
6. Spread the chips on a baking sheet and allow it to bake for 12 minutes until crisp brown.
7. Store the tortilla chips in a Ziploc bag for up to a week. Serve the tortilla chips with a serving of fresh guacamole.

#10 Carrot Apple Oatmeal Muffins

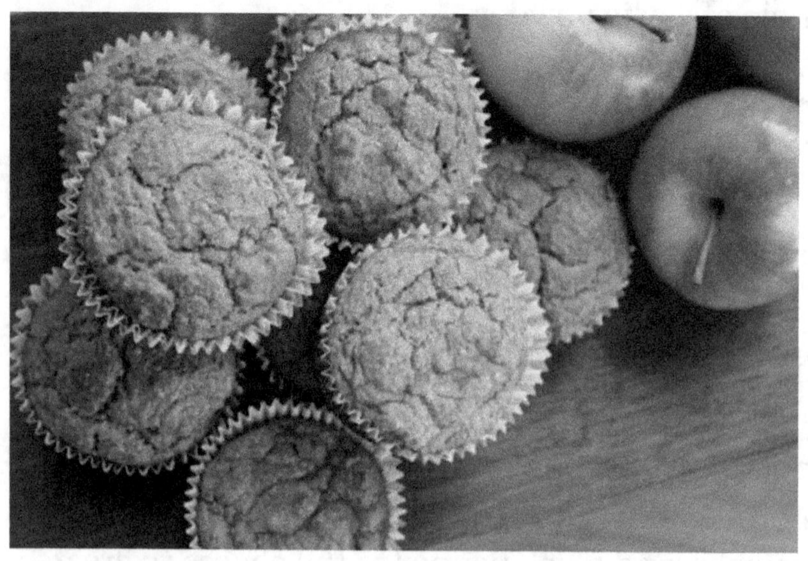

Serving size: 4+ servings

Calories: 270 (1 serving)

Preference: Dairy-free, vegetarian

Duration: 30 minutes

Ingredients:

- 2 cups of flour (all-purpose)
- 2 eggs
- 1 cup of rolled oats (gluten-free)

- 1 cup of apple (grated)
- 1 cup of carrots (grated)
- ¾ cup of brown sugar
- 2-½ tsp of baking powder
- ½ tsp of cinnamon
- ½ tsp of baking soda
- ½ tsp of ginger (ground)
- ½ tsp of vanilla extract
- ½ cup of vegetable oil
- ½ cup of almond milk

Directions:

1. Preheat the oven to 350 degrees Fahrenheit, and spray a 12-piece muffin pan with spray and cook.
2. Add the flour, baking powder, oats, sugar, and spices in a bowl and combine.
3. Add the eggs, almond milk, vegetable oil, and vanilla extract into a separate bowl and whisk everything together.
4. Add the wet ingredient mixture to the dry ingredients. Mix everything until you've reached a smooth consistency. Don't over-mix.
5. Place the batter in the muffin tin, divide evenly until the muffin tin cups are about ¾ full.
6. Place the muffins into the oven for 20 minutes. Then, remove it from the oven, allow it to cool down before removing it from the tin.
7. Place the muffins in an airtight container, and refrigerate it for up to a week.

Light and Healthy Dessert Recipes

#1 Banana Peanut Butter Ice Cream

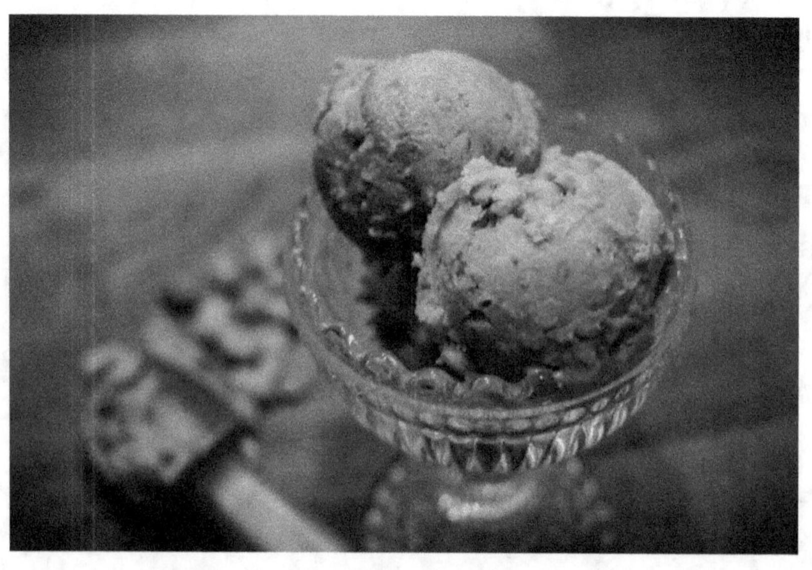

Serving size: 4+ servings

Calories: 190 (1 serving)

Preference: Gluten-free, vegetarian

Duration: 10 minutes + 1 hour in the freezer

Ingredients:

- 4 bananas (ripe, chopped frozen)

- 2 tbsps. of almond milk

- 1-2 tbsps. of peanut butter

- 1 tsp of cinnamon

- 1 tbsp. of dark chocolate

- 1 tbsp. of almonds (blanched)

- 1 tbsp. of honey

Directions:

1. Add the bananas and almond milk to a blender. Blend for 1-2 minutes.

2. Add the peanut butter, honey, and cinnamon. Blend for 1 minute.

3. Transfer the ice-cream mixture to the freezer in a freezer-proof container. Freeze it for 1 hour.

4. Serve the ice cream with 1 tbsp. of grated chocolate and blanched almonds on top.

#2 Ricotta Cannoli

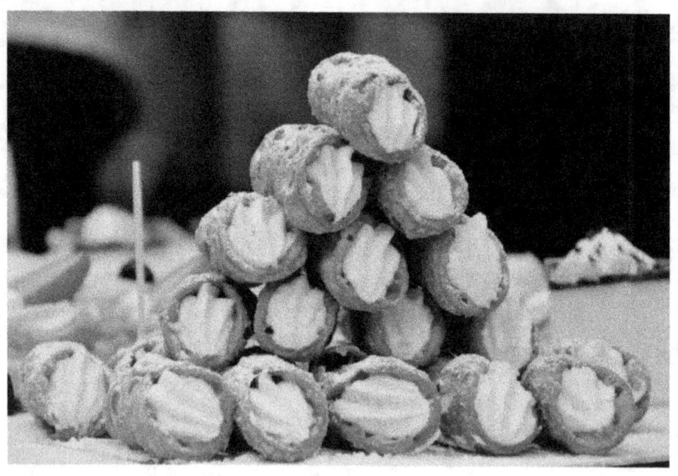

Serving size: 4+ servings

Calories: 280 (1 serving)

Preference: Vegetarian

Duration: 25 minutes

Ingredients:

- 2 egg whites
- ⅓ cup of brown sugar
- ⅓ cup of flour (all-purpose)
- 1 tbsp. of butter (melted)
- 1 tbsp. of olive oil
- 1 tsp of vanilla
- Filling: ½ cup of whipped cream, ½ cup of ricotta cheese, 3 tbsps. of cream cheese, 3 tbsps. of chocolate chips, 1 tsp of vanilla extract, 1 tsp of orange zest grated, and ½ cup of powdered sugar.

Directions:

1. Preheat the oven to 375 degrees Fahrenheit and line two baking sheets with parchment paper.
2. Add the eggs, olive oil, sugar, butter, and vanilla to a bowl, and whisk everything together.
3. Add the flour to the wet mixture, and mix it until you've reached a smooth consistency.
4. Spoon 3 tbsps. of the mixture onto the baking sheet, creating mounds about 2 inches apart.
5. Press down on the individual mounds with the back of a spoon until it reaches a size of 4 inches in diameter.
6. Bake the cookies for 8 minutes, and use a spatula to loosen them and shape it into a tube-like (cannoli) form. Allow the cookies to cool down.
7. Prepare the ricotta filling by adding the whipped cream to a mixing bowl. Whisk it until it becomes fluffy. Place the cream in the fridge until it becomes stiff.
8. Add the ricotta cheese, powdered sugar, cream cheese, orange zest, and vanilla into a separate bowl and mix the ingredients.
9. Add the cream and melted chocolate chips to the mixture (don't mix).
10. Spoon the filling inside a pastry bag and fill the cannoli shells.
11. Refrigerate the cannolis in an airtight container for up to three days.

#3 Chocolate Zucchini Muffins

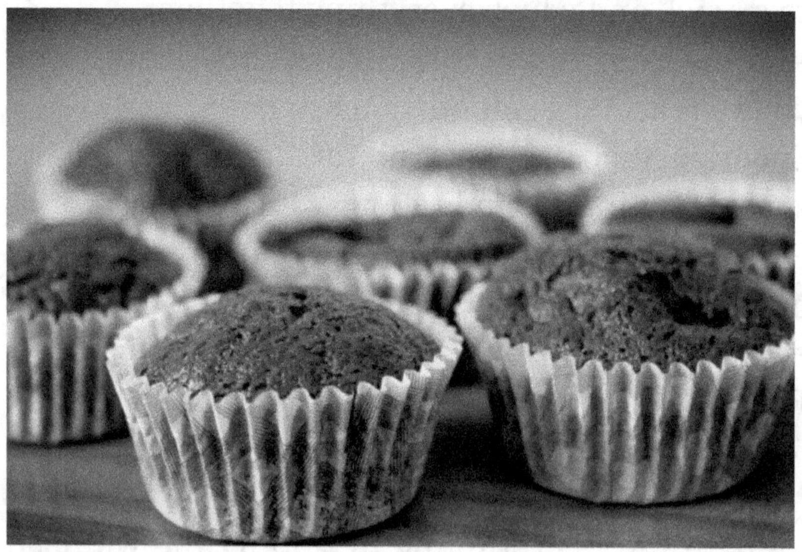

Serving size: 4+ servings

Calories: 360 (1 serving)

Preference: Vegetarian

Duration: 30 minutes

Ingredients:

- 1 cup of whole wheat flour
- 2 eggs
- 1 cup of zucchini (grated)
- ½ cup of chocolate chips
- ½ cup of cocoa powder

- ½ cup of Greek yogurt
- ⅓ cup of applesauce
- ¼ cup of honey
- ¼ cup of brown sugar
- 2 tsp of vanilla extract
- 1-½ tsp of baking powder
- ½ tsp of baking soda
- ¼ tsp of salt

<u>*Directions:*</u>

1. Preheat the oven to 350 degrees Fahrenheit, and line a muffin pan with muffin cups.
2. Combine the flour, baking powder, baking soda, cocoa, chocolate chips, and salt in a bowl.
3. Add the eggs to a second bowl, and whisk them together. Then, add the yogurt, applesauce, sugar, honey, and vanilla. Mix the ingredients until it is well combined.
4. Add the zucchini to the wet mixture.
5. Add the wet ingredients to the remaining dry ingredients. Mix everything until well combined.
6. Divide the batter between the 12 muffin cups, filling it ¾ full each. Add extra chocolate chips on top.
7. Bake the chocolate muffins in the oven for 20 minutes.
8. Store the muffins in an airtight container for up to five days.

#4 Sweet Cherry Crisp

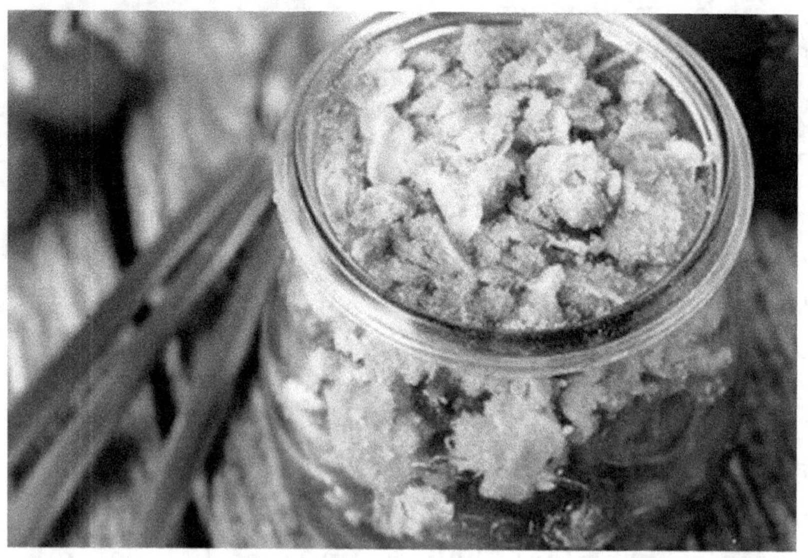

Serving size: 4 servings

Calories: 420 (1 serving)

Preference: Dairy-free, vegetarian

Duration: 30 minutes

Ingredients:

- 6 cups of cherries (pitted and halved)
- 2 tbsps. lemon juice
- 2 tbsps. of honey

- 1 tsp of lemon zest
- 2 tbsps. of arrowroot starch
- 1 tsp of vanilla extract
- ¼ tsp salt
- Crisp/topping: 1-½ cups of raw almonds, 1 cup of rolled oats, 2 tbsps. of honey, 1 tbsp. of coconut oil (melted), 2 tsp of cinnamon, ¼ tsp of salt

Directions:

1. Preheat the oven to 350 degrees Fahrenheit and grease four ramekins with coconut oil.
2. Combine the cherries, honey, arrowroot starch, lemon juice, zest, and salt in a bowl.
3. For the crisp, add the almonds, oats, honey, cinnamon, salt, and coconut oil to a separate bowl and mix it.
4. Add the cherry mixture to the ramekins, dividing it evenly and placing it at the bottom of the dishes. Add the crisp mixture on top.
5. Place the ramekins on a baking sheet on parchment paper in the oven. Allow it to bake for 20 minutes. Allow it to cool down after removing it from the oven.
6. Add a dollop of Greek yogurt on top.
7. Serve immediately or cover the ramekins with plastic wrap. Place it in the refrigerator for up to two days.

#5 Healthy Fudge

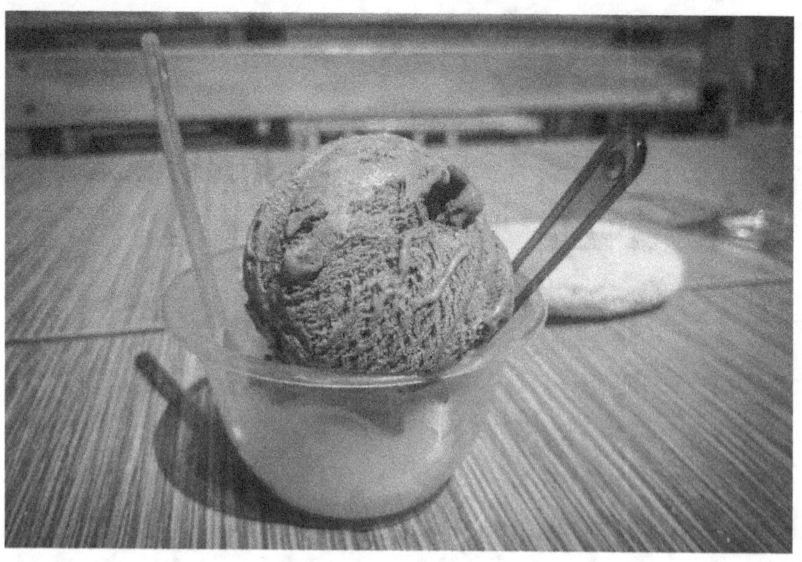

Serving size: 4+ servings

Calories: 340 (1 serving)

Preference: Gluten-free, dairy-free, vegetarian

Duration: 5 minutes +4 hours freezer

Ingredients:

- 1 13.5 oz of coconut milk (can)

- ½ cup of cocoa powder

- ⅓ cup of honey

- 2 tsp vanilla extract

Directions:

1. Add all the ingredients to a blender. Blend until you've reached a smooth consistency.

2. Add the mixture into a mold, and freeze it for 4 hours.

3. Remove the fudge from the mold once it is set, and store it in an airtight container for five to seven days.

#6 Frozen Yogurt

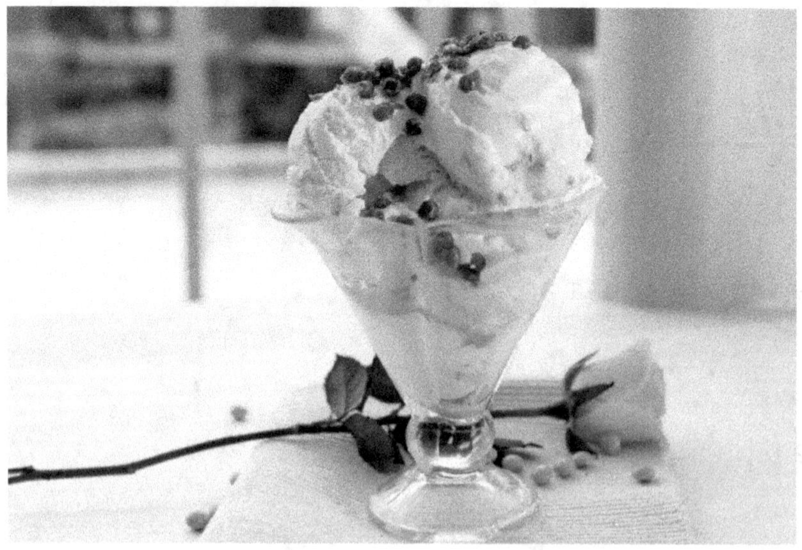

Serving size: 4 servings

Calories: 90 (1 serving)

Preference: Gluten-free, vegetarian

Duration: 10 minutes

Ingredients:

- 2 bananas (ripe and sliced)

- ¾ cup of Greek yogurt

- 2 tsp of honey

Directions:

1. Add the frozen bananas to a blender. Then add the dark cocoa powder, Greek yogurt, and honey. Blend the ingredients until you've reached a smooth consistency.

2. Serve the frozen yogurt immediately or place it in an airtight container in the freezer until ready to serve. Store the frozen yogurt in the freezer for up to a month.

#7 Peanut Butter Cookies

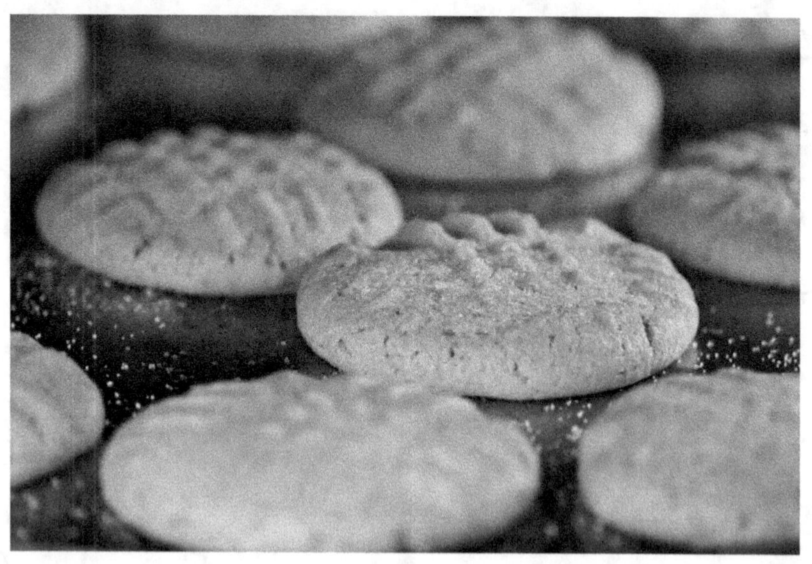

Serving size: 4+ servings

Calories: 300 (1 serving)

Preference: Dairy-free, vegetarian

Duration: 20 minutes

Ingredients:

- 1 cup of peanut butter
- ⅔ cups of brown sugar
- ½ cup of baking flour
- ¼ cup of shredded coconut
- 2 eggs

Directions:

1. Preheat the oven to 350 degrees Fahrenheit and line a baking sheet with parchment paper.
2. Add the peanut butter, sugar, flour, coconut, and eggs in a bowl. Mix the ingredients.
3. Scoop 2 tbsp of the cookie batter. Roll it into a bowl, and place it on the baking sheet. Flatten the balls using your palms and place them on the cookie sheet. Repeat this step until the dough is finished.
4. Use a fork to press down on each cookie, and transfer the cookie sheet to the oven. Bake the cookies for 10 minutes.
5. Remove the cookies from the oven, allow it to cool down.
6. Store it in Ziploc bags for up to a week.

#8 Chia Pudding

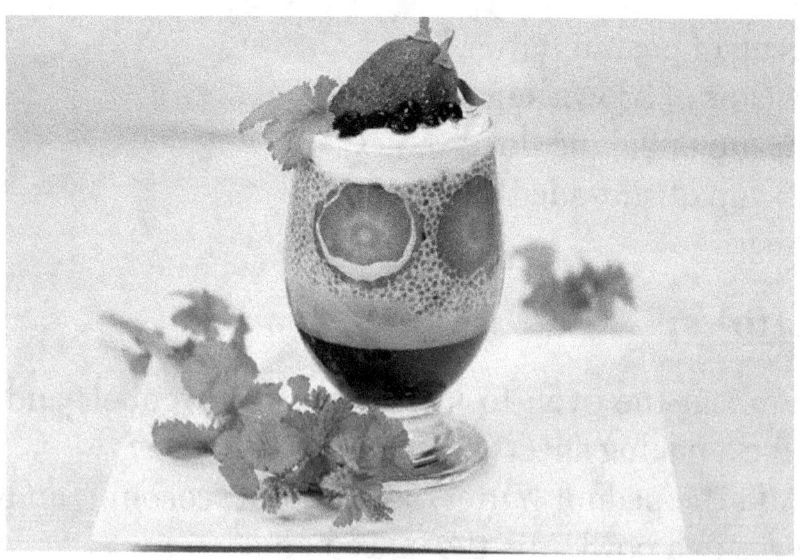

Serving size: 4 servings

Calories: 150 (1 serving)

Preference: Gluten-free, dairy-free, vegetarian

Duration: 5-10 minutes

Ingredients:

- 2 cups of almond milk

- 8 tbsps. of chia seeds

- 4 tsp of honey

- 1 cup of strawberries (sliced)

Directions:

1. Divide the ingredients and pour them into four mason jars. Mix everything well.

2. Cover the jar. Store it in the refrigerator for 2 hours, and serve cold. The chia pudding can be stored in the refrigerator for up to two days.

#9 Cashew Bars

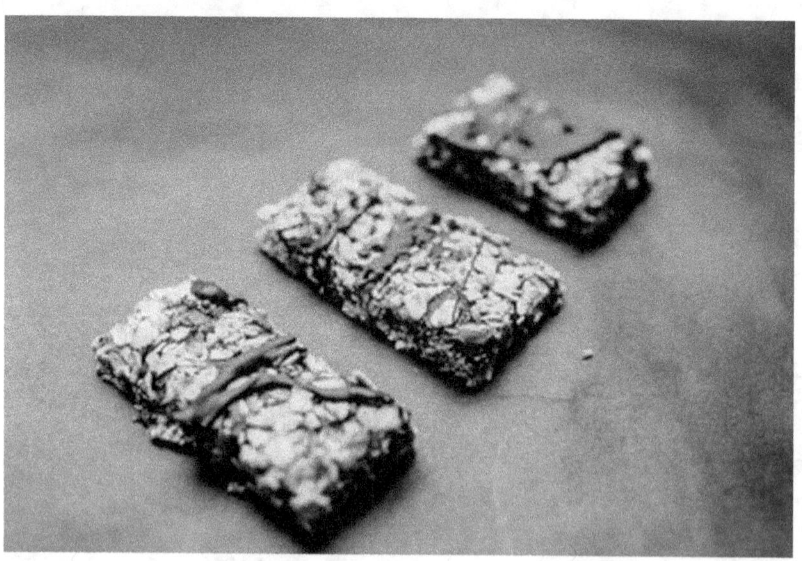

Serving size: 4+ servings

Calories: 580 (1 serving)

Preference: Gluten-free, vegetarian

Duration: 25 minutes

<u>*Ingredients:*</u>

- 8 dates (pitted)
- 1 cup of cashews (roasted)
- ¾ cup of tahini
- 2 tsp of vanilla extract
- 12 pieces of dark chocolate
- ¼ cup of sesame seeds
- ¼ cup of cranberries

<u>*Directions:*</u>

1. Place parchment paper into a square baking dish.
2. Add the dates, tahini, vanilla extract, and cashews to a food processor. Mix everything for 4 minutes, or until well combined. Transfer the mixture to the freezer for 30 minutes.
3. Place chocolate in the microwave and allow it to melt until smooth. Then, allow it to cool for 10 minutes. Cut the bars into large squares, whichever the number of servings you want.
4. Place it in the fridge between two pieces of parchment paper, allowing the chocolate to set for about 10 minutes.
5. Store it in the fridge in an airtight container for up to a week.

#10 Chocolate Brownies

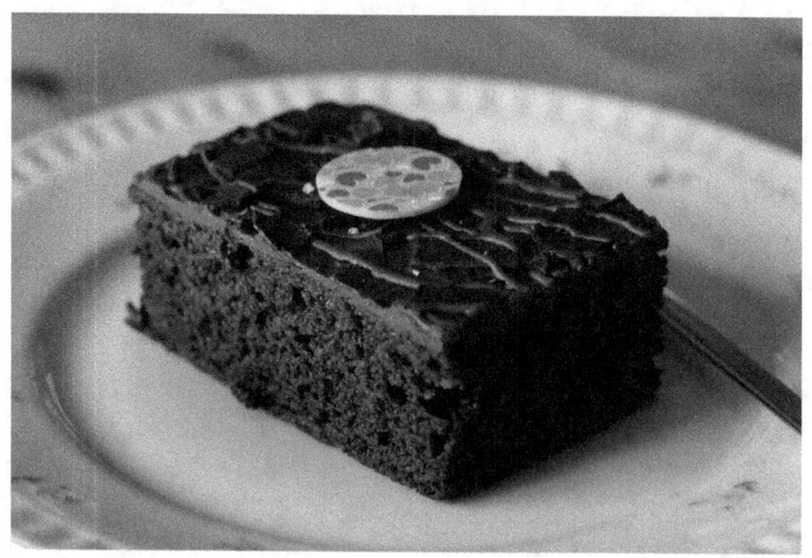

Serving size: 4+ servings

Calories: 250 (1 serving)

Preference: Vegetarian

Duration: 30 minutes + 6 hrs set time

Ingredients:

- 2 egg whites
- ¼ cup of Greek yogurt
- ½ cup of coconut sugar
- ¾ cup of cocoa powder
- ¾ cup of whole wheat flour

- 6 tbsps. of almond milk
- 3 tbsps. of dark chocolate (chopped)
- 1 tbsp. of coconut oil (melted)
- 1 tsp of vanilla extract
- ¼ tsp of baking powder
- ¼ tsp of salt

Directions:

1. Preheat the oven to 300 degrees Fahrenheit and coat a square baking dish with cooking spray.
2. Add the egg whites, vanilla, salt, and butter to a bowl and whisk the ingredients together. Then, add the Greek yogurt. Mix the ingredients until it is lump-free. Add the coconut sugar, almond milk, cocoa powder, and baking powder.
3. Finally, add the flour and mix the batter well. Once mixed, add the dark chocolate.
4. Add the butter to the dish, and add added dark chocolate on top.
5. Bake the batter for 15 minutes.
6. Once done, remove it from the oven and allow it to cool and set at room temperature for 6 hours.
7. Serve immediately, or store the brownies between two pieces of parchment paper in the refrigerator, in an airtight container.

#11 Quinoa Peanut Brittle

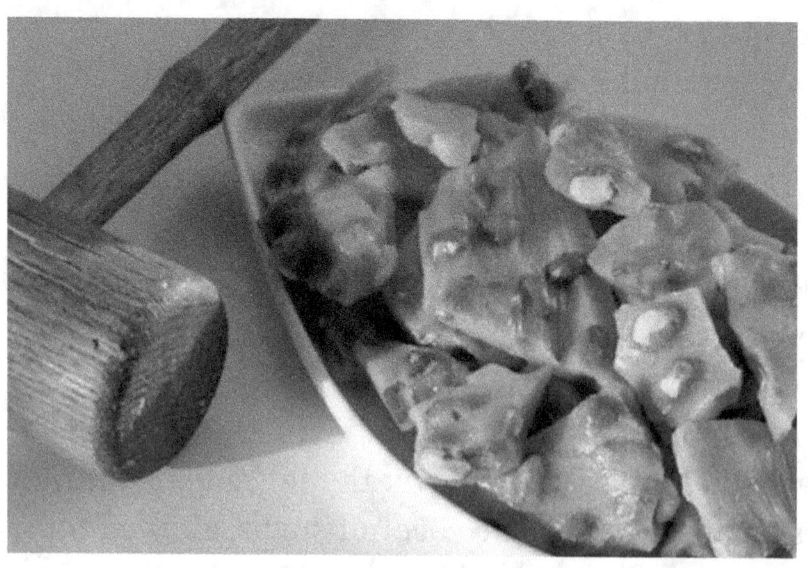

Serving size: 4+ servings

Calories: 380 (1 serving)

Preference: Gluten-free, dairy-free, vegetarian

Duration: 25 minutes

Ingredients:

- ½ cup of quinoa
- ¾ cup of peanuts (raw and chopped)

- ⅔ cup of honey
- ⅓ cup of rolled oats (gluten-free)
- 2 tbsps. of brown sugar
- 2 tbsps. of chia seeds
- 2 tbsps. of coconut oil (melted)
- ½ tsp of vanilla extract
- ⅛ tsp of Himalayan salt

Directions:

1. Preheat the oven to 325 degrees Fahrenheit and line a baking sheet with parchment paper.
2. Combine the quinoa (uncooked), raw peanuts, brown sugar, rolled oats, chia seeds, and Himalayan salt in a bowl. Stir the ingredients together until well combined.
3. Add melted vanilla extract, honey, and coconut oil to a separate bowl and mix everything. Combine with the dry mixture, and mix once more.
4. Transfer the mixture to the baking sheet, spreading it evenly.
5. Allow it to bake in the oven for 15 minutes, and then remove it.
6. Allow the peanut brittle to cool down before cutting or breaking it up into pieces.
7. Store the peanut brittle in a container in a Ziploc bag at room temperature for five to seven days.

Chapter 3: Weekly Meal Plans and Shopping Lists

Week 1 + Shopping List

Monday 1630 (kcal)

Breakfast: Egg Salad Sandwiches

Snack: Paleo Granola

Lunch: Creamy Tofu Salad

Dinner: Sesame Noodles

Dessert: Chia Pudding

Tuesday 1650(kcal)

Breakfast: Banana Blueberry Protein Muffins

Snack: Wholesome Crackers

Lunch: Vegetable Nourish Jars

Dinner: Turkey Breasts and Vegetables

Dessert: Sweet Cherry Crisp

Wednesday 1630 (kcal)

Breakfast: Egg Salad Sandwiches

Snack: Paleo Granola

Lunch: Creamy Tofu Salad

Dinner: Sesame Noodles

Dessert: Chia Pudding

Thursday 1660 (kcal)

Breakfast: Peanut Butter Bites

Snack: Avocado Chips

Lunch: Vegetable Nourish Jars

Dinner: Turkey Breasts and Vegetables

Dessert: Chocolate Zucchini Muffins

Friday 1695 (kcal)

Breakfast: Pumpkin Glow Smoothie

Snack: Tortilla Chips with Guacamole

Lunch: Mexican Pasta Salad

Dinner: Cauliflower Tacos

Dessert: Frozen Yogurt

Saturday 1620 (kcal)

Breakfast: Banana Blueberry Protein Muffins

Snack: Wholesome Crackers

Lunch: Teriyaki Chicken

Dinner: Red Lentil Dal

Dessert: Sweet Cherry Crips

Sunday 1705 (kcal)

Breakfast: Pumpkin Glow Smoothie

Snack: Tortilla Chips with Guacamole

Lunch: Mexican Pasta Salad

Dinner: Couscous Salad

Dessert: Chocolate Zucchini Muffins

Shopping List

Pantry:

Gluten-free bread - 16 slices
Corn tortillas (plantain) – 12

Vanilla extract
Brown sugar
Chocolate chips - 1 ½ cup
Baking soda – 1 ½ tsp
Almond flour - 5 cups
Coconut flour - 1 cup
Flaxseed meal (ground) - 2 tsp
Whole-wheat flour - 2 cup
Arrowroot starch - 4 tbsp
Cocoa powder - 1 cup
Coconut flakes - 1 cup
Baking powder - 3 tsp

Flax seeds (ground) - ½ cup
Chia seeds - 24 tsp
Pumpkin seeds - 1 cup
Flaxseeds - 0.5 cup
Sunflower seeds - 0.5 cup
Poppy seeds - 2 tsp

Sesame seeds - 1 tsp

....

Pecan nuts - 3 cup
Almonds - 2 ¼ cup
Cashews - 1 cup

....

Black beans 1 cup
Pure pumpkin (canned) - 8 tbsp
Corn 1 cup
Olives (halved) - 5 oz
Cherry tomatoes - one 15-oz can

....

Pasta (gluten-free) - 20 oz
Rolled oats (gluten-free) - 3 cup
Couscous (packages) - 2 4.7-oz
Quinoa – 1 ½ cup (cooked)
Red lentils - 2 cups
Chickpeas - (1 can) 15 oz

....

Hummus (plain) - 8 tsp
Guacamole (store-bought) - 2 cup

....

Honey
Agave nectar - 2 tbsp
Maple syrup - 1 tbsp

Applesauce - ½ cup

Apple cider vinegar
Rice wine vinegar

Oils/sauces/seasonings:
Oil
Olive oil
Coconut oil
Sesame oil
Avocado oil
Peanut butter
Italian seasoning
Salsa 1 cup
Soy sauce (low-sodium)
Dijon mustard

Spices:
Salt
Himalayan salt
Onion powder
Garlic powder
Black pepper
Cayenne pepper
Red chili flakes

Paprika

Cinnamon
Nutmeg
Thyme
Rosemary (chopped)
Cumin
Oregano
Basil
Parsley
Thyme
Cilantro
Turmeric
Curry powder

Dairy/dairy-alternatives:
Greek yogurt - 7 cups
Almond milk - 5 ½ cups
Mozzarella cheese (grated) - 5 cups
Soft tofu - 2 lb
Cashew milk - 1 cup
Edamame - ¼ cup
Coconut milk - 1 oz

Protein:
Eggs - 22

Lean turkey - 10 strips
Chicken breasts - 3
Turkey breasts - 32 oz
Salami (chopped) - 5 oz

Fruit:
Blueberries - 1 cup
Strawberries - 4 cups
Cherries - 12 cups
Cranberries - 2 cups

Lemon - 2
Lime - 2
Apple - 2
Bananas - 14
Pineapple (chopped) - ¼ cup

Vegetables:
Green onion - 5 cups
Celery stalks - 10 stalks
Large lettuce leaves - 8
Romaine lettuce leaves - 16
Red cabbage (sliced) - ¼ cup

Cauliflower heads (chopped) - 2

Broccoli - 6 cups

Baby carrots - 5 cups
Cherry tomatoes (halved) - 2 cups
Zucchini (grated) - 2 cup
Potatoes (peeled, washed, and chopped) - 4 cups

Chipotle peppers - 2 whole
Green bell pepper - 1
Red bell peppers - 6 cups

Avocado (large) - 2
Pure pumpkin (canned) - 8 tbsp
Baby marrow (chopped) - 5 cups
Garlic cloves - 7

Monday 1630 (kcal)

Breakfast: Breakfast Burritos

Snack: Avocado chips

Lunch: Steak Cobb Salad

Dinner: Red Lentil Dal

Dessert: Healthy Fudge

Tuesday 1560 (kcal)

Breakfast: Tropical Smoothie Bowl

Snack: Chocolate Bark

Lunch: Teriyaki Chicken

Dinner: Spicy Quinoa Jars

Dessert: Ricotta Cannoli

Wednesday 1680 (kcal)

Breakfast: Tropical Smoothie Bowl

Snack: Avocado chips

Lunch: Steak Cobb Salad

Dinner: Cauliflower Tacos

Dessert: Healthy Fudge

Thursday 1680 (kcal)

Breakfast: Egg Salad Sandwiches

Snack: Paleo Granola

Lunch: Salmon Salad

Dinner: Cauliflower Tacos

Dessert: Frozen Yogurt

Friday 1690 (kcal)

Breakfast: Honey Granola and Greek Yogurt

Snack: Chocolate Bark

Lunch: Teriyaki Chicken

Dinner: Buffalo Tofu Jars

Dessert: Ricotta Cannoli

Saturday 1680 (kcal)

Breakfast: Blueberry-Coconut Chia Jars

Snack: Tortilla Chips with Guacamole

Lunch: Salmon Salad

Dinner: Sesame Noodles

Dessert: Chocolate Brownies

Sunday 1690 (kcal)

Breakfast: Honey Granola and Greek Yogurt

Snack: Wholesome Crackers

Lunch: French Sandwiches

Dinner: Buffalo Tofu Jars

Dessert: Chocolate Brownies

Shopping List

Pantry:

Whole-wheat tortillas (large) - 4
Gluten-free bread - 8 slices
Pretzels (chopped) - 1 cup
Corn tortillas (plantain) – 24

Black beans - 15 oz. + 1 cup
15-oz can of cherry tomatoes - 2
Corn - 1 cup

Raisins - 1 cup
Almonds - 2 cups
Mixed nuts - 2 cups
Pistachios - 0.5 cup
Pecan nuts - 3 cups

Almond flour - 4 cups
Coconut flour - ½ cup
Flaxseeds meal (ground) - 1 tsp
Flour (all-purpose) - 0.5 cup
Whole-wheat flour - 1.5 cups
Hummus (plain) - 4 tsp

Guacamole (store-bought) - 1 cup
Tahini - ¼ cup

Rolled oats (gluten-free) - 10 cups
Red lentils (dried) - 2 cups
Quinoa (cooked) - 4-½ cups
Stir fry noodles (whole wheat) - 6 oz.

Honey - 5 cups
Maple syrup - 2 tbsp.

Chia seeds - 4 tbsp.
Pumpkin seeds - ½ cup
Flaxseeds - ¼ cup
Sunflower seeds - ¼ cup
Sesame seeds - 3.5 tsp

Dark choc chips (12 oz, melted) - 5 bags
Coconut flakes - 1 cup
Brown sugar
Coconut sugar - 1 cup
Powdered sugar - 1 cup
Whipped cream - 1 cup
Baking powder

Oils/sauces/seasonings:

Butter - 6 tbsp
Olive oil
Coconut oil - 7 tbsp
Sesame oil - 3 tsp
Avocado oil - 8 tbsp

Salsa - ½ cup
Soy sauce (low-sodium) 1 cup
Rice vinegar
Italian seasoning - 1 tsp
Worcestershire sauce
Buffalo sauce (vegan) - 1 cup

Spices:

Black pepper
Cayenne pepper
Chili flakes
Paprika

Salt
Himalayan salt
Kosher salt

Cinnamon

Thyme
Onion powder
Garlic powder
Rosemary
Turmeric
Cumin
Ginger
Cilantro
Curry powder
Coriander
Basil

Nutmeg
Vanilla extract
Vanilla
Cocoa powder

Dairy/non-dairy alternatives:
Mozzarella cheese - 4.5 cups
Edamame - 2.5 cups
Feta cheese - 1 cup
Tofu (firm and cubed) - 4 cups
Ricotta cheese - 1 cup
Cream cheese - 6 tbsp
Almond milk - 5 cups

Coconut milk (can) - 4 13.5 oz
Greek yogurt - 9 cups

Protein:
Eggs - 23
Steak (lean cut) - 2 oz
Chicken breasts (halved) - 3
Chicken breast (cooked and chopped) - 1 lb

Fruit:
Bananas -6
Mango - 4 cups
Pineapple - 2.5 cups
Kiwis - 4
Orange - 1
Mango - 1
Lemon - 5
Lime – 4

Blueberries - 2 cups
Mixed berries - 4 cups
Cranberries - 1 cup

Vegetables:
Large lettuce leaves - 4
Baby spinach - 12 cups
Celery - 2 stalks + 4 cups
Romaine lettuce heads (chopped) - 2
Romaine lettuce (shredded) - 16 cups

Avocado - 7
Cherry tomatoes - 1 cup
Rosa tomatoes - 6 cups
Broccoli - 6 cups
Cauliflower heads (chopped) - 4
Red cabbage - 0.5 cup
Cucumbers - 2

Baby carrots - 2 cups
Carrots - 4 cups

Jalapeno - 1
Whole chipotle peppers – 4

Onion - ½
Green onion - 2 cups
Spring onion (small and sliced) - 2
Garlic cloves - 11

Week 3 + Shopping List

Monday 1605 (kcal)

Breakfast: Get-Your-Greens Sweet Potato Frittata

Snack: Carrot Apple Oatmeal Muffins

Lunch: Chicken and Avocado Burritos

Dinner: Spaghetti Squash Boats

Dessert: Banana Peanut Butter Ice Cream

Tuesday 1650 (kcal)

Breakfast: Sweet Vitamin-Kick Walnut Oatmeal

Snack: Deviled Eggs with Hummus

Lunch: Vegetable Nourish Jars

Dinner: Honey Sriracha Meatballs

Dessert: Sweet Cherry Crisp

Wednesday 1635 (kcal)

Breakfast: Get-Your-Greens Sweet Potato Frittata

Snack: Sweet and Salty Nuts

Lunch: Salmon Salad

Dinner: Couscous Salad

Dessert: Banana Peanut Butter Ice Cream

Thursday 1655 (kcal)

Breakfast: Pumpkin Glow Smoothie

Snack: Protein Balls

Lunch: Chicken Avocado Burritos

Dinner: Honey Sriracha Meatballs

Dessert: Peanut Butter Cookies

Friday 1610 (kcal)

Breakfast: Blueberry Coconut Chia Jars

Snack: Protein Balls

Lunch: Cauliflower Casserole with Mushrooms and Cheese

Dinner: Spaghetti Squash Boats

Dessert: Carrot Apple Oatmeal Muffins

Saturday 1610 (kcal)

Breakfast: Sweet Vitamin-Kick Walnut Oatmeal

Snack: Chocolate-Dipped Clementines

Lunch: Protein Lettuce Wraps

Dinner: Spicy Chicken and Rice

Dessert: Quinoa Peanut Brittle

<u>Sunday 1650 (kcal)</u>

Breakfast: Blueberry Coconut Chia Jars

Snack: Protein Balls

Lunch: Cauliflower Casserole with Mushrooms and Cheese

Dinner: Red Lentil Dal

Dessert: Chocolate Zucchini Muffins

Shopping List

Pantry:

Whole-wheat tortillas – 8

Rolled oats (gluten-free) – 11 cups
Quinoa – 2-½ cups
Macaroni (gluten-free) -8 oz
Red lentils – 3 cups
Couscous (packages) - 2 4.7-oz
Brown rice – 1 cup

Honey – 5 cups

Walnuts – 2 cups
Raw almonds – 5 cups
Peanuts - ¾ cup

Vanilla extract
Brown sugar
Coconut sugar - ½ cup
Baking powder
Baking soda
Cocoa powder -2 cups

Arrowroot starch – 2 tbsp
Nutritional yeast - ½ cup
Chocolate chips – 1 ½ cups
Dark chocolate - 5 tbsp
Breadcrumbs (whole wheat)

Pure pumpkin (canned) - 8 tbsp
Hummus (smooth) – 1 ½ cups
Dijon mustard

Chia seeds – 18 tbsp
Flaxseeds - 6 tbsp

Diced tomatoes (can) – 4

15 oz. of chickpeas (can) – 1
Black beans - 1 14 oz

Flour (all-purpose) – 3 cups
Baking flour - ½ cup
Whole wheat flour – 1 ¾ cups

Apple cider vinegar – 3 tbsp
Rice vinegar - 1-½ tbsp.
Red wine vinegar - ⅓ cup

Oils/sauces/seasonings

Peanut butter – 4 cups
Olive oil
Extra-virgin olive oil
Vegetable oil
Coconut oil
Sesame oil

Salsa – 14 oz.+ ½ cup
Sriracha - ¼ cup
Tahini – 1 tbsp
Italian seasoning – 2 tbsp
Soy sauce (low-sodium) – 2 ½ tbsp
Applesauce - ⅓ cup

Spices:
Garlic powder
Ginger powder
Chili powder
Curry powder

Black pepper
Cayenne pepper
Paprika

Salt
Himalayan salt
Kosher salt
Sea salt

··

Cinnamon
Nutmeg
Thyme
Basil
Oregano
Red chili flakes
Turmeric
Cumin

Dairy/non-dairy alternatives:
Mozzarella cheese 5oz + 3.5 cups
Edamame – 1 cup
Cheddar cheese – 16 oz

··

Greek yogurt – 3 cups
Almond milk- 6 cups
Coconut milk – 1 oz + 6 cups
Nut milk - 6 tbsp
Cashew milk – 6 cups

Protein:

Eggs 37

Chicken -2 oz + 1 lb

Salmon fillets - 2 6-oz

Shrimp (peeled and deveined) – 2lb

Turkey (ground) – 2 lb

Salami (chopped) -5 oz

Fruit:

Blueberries – 2 cups

Cherries – 6 cups

Pineapple (chopped) – 4 cups

Clementine oranges - 5

Lemon – 2

Lime – 1

Orange - 1

Bananas – 12

Apple – 1 cup

Shredded coconut - 2 cup

Ginger (grated) - 3 piece

Vegetables:

Sweet potato (washed, peeled, and cubed) - 5 cups

Carrots – 1 cup

Baby carrots – 2 cups
Cucumber – 1 cup
Cherry tomatoes – 4 cup
Brown mushrooms - 2 lb.
Cauliflower florets – 6 cups
Spaghetti squash (halved) – 4
Zucchini – 1 cup

....

Avocado – 4
Olives (halved) – 5 oz.

....

Kale (washed and chopped) 4 cups
Butter lettuce leaves (large) -16
Cabbage (purple and chopped) – 1 cup
Lettuce (chopped) – 4 cups
Fresh parsley - ¼ cup
Cilantro (fresh) – 1 tbsp

....

Red bell pepper – 1
Green bell pepper – 1

....

Red onion (diced) - ½ cup
Onion – 3
Pickled onions - ¼ cup
Garlic – 9 cloves

Conclusion

This Healthy Meal Planning for Beginners guide is convenient for any type of individual. It can change your perspective on healthy food options and drive you to become excited about preparing three- to seven-days' worth of meals each week. Since all the recipes included in this guide are extremely delicious, easy to make, and nutritious, it can help you stay motivated on your health and weight loss journey without it even feeling like you're punishing yourself or following a strict diet. This adds to the effectiveness of meal planning as a means to promote weight loss and boost your health, all at the expense of convenience.

References

10 healthy eating rules from a nutritionist. (2018). Retrieved from Onemedical.com website: https://www.onemedical.com/blog/eat-well/healthy-eating-checklist

20+ Healthy Meal Prep Lunch Ideas for Work - The Girl on Bloor. (2020, January 2). Retrieved January 21, 2020, from The Girl on Bloor website: https://thegirlonbloor.com/20-easy-healthy-meal-prep-lunch-ideas-for-work/

29 Healthy Snacks That Can Help You Lose Weight. (2016). Retrieved from Healthline website: https://www.healthline.com/nutrition/29-healthy-snacks-for-weight-loss

36+ Healthy Breakfast Meal Prep Ideas. (2016, September 10). Retrieved January 21, 2020, from Sweet Peas and Saffron website: https://sweetpeasandsaffron.com/28-healthy-meal-prep-breakfast-ideas/

Cohen, L. (2018, February 7). 55 Quick and Easy Healthy Breakfasts for Your Busiest Mornings. Retrieved January 21, 2020, from Good Housekeeping website: https://www.goodhousekeeping.com/food-recipes/easy/g871/quick-breakfasts/?slide=1

Country Living Staff. (2017, April 28). 40 Best Healthy Desserts That Are Totally Guilt-Free. Retrieved January 24, 2020, from Country Living website: https://www.countryliving.com/food-drinks/g1331/healthy-desserts/?slide=6

Flager, M. (2018, March 14). 42 Healthy Snacks That Are WAY Better Than Anything In A Vending Machine. Retrieved from Delish website: https://www.delish.com/cooking/nutrition/g600/healthy-snacks-for-work/

Fulcher, A. (2019, July 14). 20 Healthy Dinners You Can Meal Prep on Sunday. Retrieved January 23, 2020, from The

Everygirl website: https://theeverygirl.com/20-healthy-dinners-you-can-meal-prep-on-sunday/

Fulcher, A. (2018, May 13). 20 Lunches You Can Meal Prep on Sunday. Retrieved January 21, 2020, from The Everygirl website: https://theeverygirl.com/20-lunches-you-can-meal-prep-on-sunday/

Hali Bey Ramdene. (2017, March 19). The Beginner's Guide to Meal Planning: What to Know, How to Succeed, and What to Skip. Retrieved December 16, 2019, from Kitchn website: https://www.thekitchn.com/the-beginners-guide-to-meal-planning-what-to-know-how-to-succeed-and-what-to-skip-242413

Halse, H. (2010, July 20). Formula for Caloric Intake. Retrieved January 20, 2020, from LIVESTRONG.COM website: https://www.livestrong.com/article/178764-caloric-intake-formula/

https://www.facebook.com/GatheringDreamsBlog. (2019, March). 25 Healthy Meal Prep Ideas To Simplify Your Life. Retrieved January 23, 2020, from Gathering Dreams website: https://gatheringdreams.com/easy-healthy-meal-prep-ideas-30-minutes/

Institute of Medicine (US) Subcommittee on Interpretation and Uses of Dietary Reference Intakes, & Institute of Medicine (US) Standing Committee on the Scientific Evaluation of Dietary Reference Intakes. (2012). Introduction to Dietary Planning. Retrieved January 20, 2020, from Nih.gov website: https://www.ncbi.nlm.nih.gov/books/NBK221366/

Sonalie Figueiras. (2015, May 4). Green Queen Health: The 7 Golden Rules Of Healthy Eating (That Anyone Can Follow). Retrieved January 20, 2020, from Green Queen website: https://www.greenqueen.com.hk/the-7-golden-rules-of-healthy-eating-that-anyone-can-follow/

Thank You

For Reading!

Please,

Leave Me Your

Review!